Get Healthy

An Easy Way to Eat
Satisfying, High-Fiber Meals
and Stay Motivated

Christopher Crennen

Warnings and Disclaimers

This publication is not intended as a substitute for medical advice from a physician. Because of your unique medical condition, the diet recommended in this publication may not be appropriate for you. The author disclaims responsibility for adverse health outcomes and recommends regular medical checkups to monitor your health. Consult your doctor before making dietary or exercise changes.

If you have a medical condition or are taking any medicines, it is especially important to work closely with your doctor. For example, if you are taking medication for high blood pressure or for diabetes, a whole-food, plant-based diet may greatly reduce the amount of medication you need. Failure to adjust your medication can be very dangerous resulting in low blood pressure or low blood glucose. Be sure to consult regularly and frequently with your doctor and monitor your numbers at home to make sure the amount and type of medication you are taking is correct.

As another example if you are taking Coumadin (the blood thinner warfarin), foods on the diet that are high in vitamin K (for example, blueberries, carrots, cauliflower, green beans, cabbage and peas) may reduce the effectiveness of the blood thinner. Consult your doctor about how dietary changes will affect any medications you are taking.

If a vegan diet (no meat, dairy or animal foods) is eaten, a vitamin b12 supplement is needed to avoid potentially severe health consequences.

Contents

Introduction

The modern diet is not a healthy diet. An amazing sixty percent of calories in the U.S. diet are from added fats and oils (26%), white flour and other refined grains (19%) and added sugars (15%).

Obesity, type 2 diabetes and other chronic diseases have followed the adoption of this modern diet in countries around the world.

Get Healthy provides a simple, convenient way to adopt a high-fiber, whole-food, plant-based diet and a way to stay motivated until the diet becomes your routine and automatic way of eating.

Obesity and Diabetes

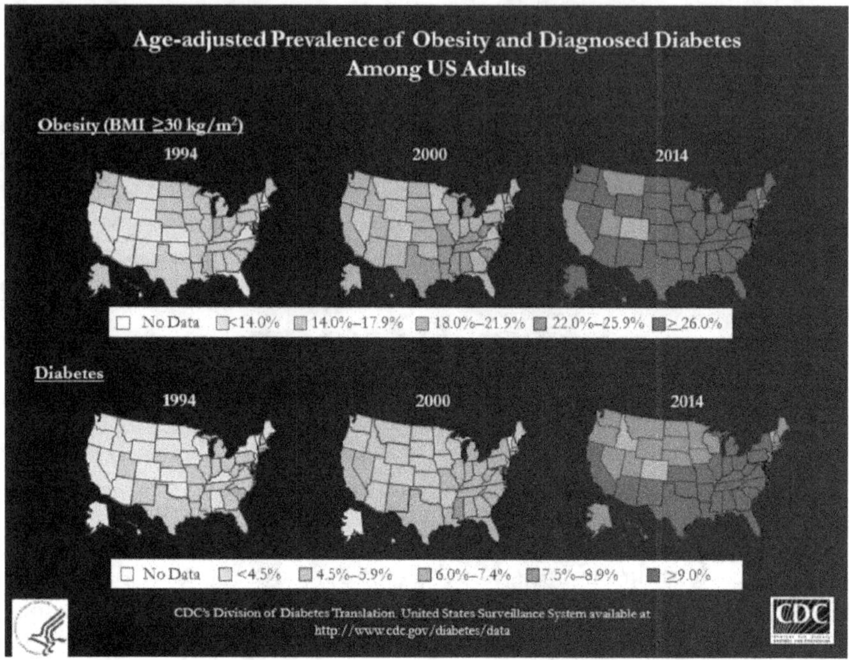

As shown on the CDC map above, epidemics of obesity and type 2 diabetes have afflicted the United States in recent decades.

The CDC reports that 39.6% of U.S. adults were obese in 2016 and that 9.4% of the U.S. population had diabetes in 2015. What has caused this alarming explosion of obesity and diabetes? One critical factor is government regulation of healthcare and food which have had severe unintended consequences.

Prior to the adoption of Medicare and Medicaid in 1965, most healthcare insurance was medically underwritten. Overweight and diabetic people were charged more for insurance than people in good health.

State and federal regulation of health insurance have increasingly prevented health insurance companies from charging people with pre-existing conditions such as high cholesterol, high blood sugar and other health risks more than healthy insureds. Removing the financial incentives of a free market has had dire consequences for the health of Americans.

Medicare currently pays out an average of over $1000 per month per beneficiary, over twice as much as most other industrialized countries. If this $1000 was paid directly to beneficiaries instead of to doctors, hospitals and pharmaceutical companies, the vast majority of beneficiaries could afford good health coverage in a free competitive market with money to spare.

The savings and innovation in American healthcare would be amazing. Only a small minority would need to depend on welfare programs such as Medicaid. Unfortunately the lobbying power of doctors, hospitals and pharmaceutical companies at both the state and federal levels makes a free market solution unlikely.

However, this book is not about political solutions to the obesity and diabetes epidemics. Instead this book is a simple, easy way that individuals can adopt a healthy, high-fiber, whole-food, plant-based diet.

Why Diets Fail

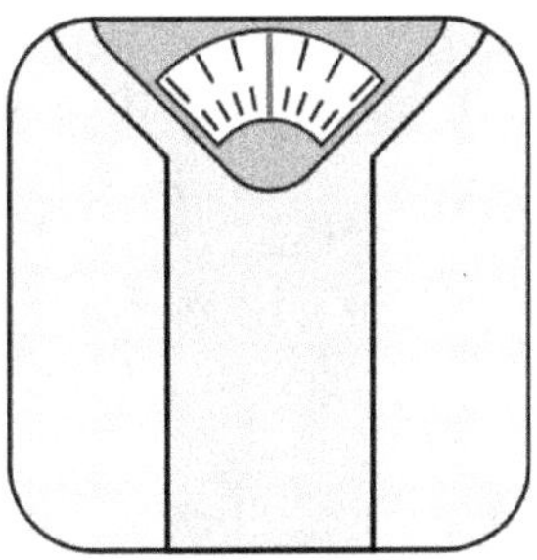

While most diets fail, evidence from the National Weight Control Registry shows that long-term weight loss is possible.

Three reasons that diets fail are:

(1) Eating unhealthy food,

(2) Failing to stay motivated, and

(3) Inconvenient, time-consuming meals.

The first three chapters of this book address the three reasons that diets often fail.

Chapter 1 on Good Food discusses the types of food to eat for permanent weight loss and good health. Many people, even the obese and diabetic, believe they eat a healthy diet. Many believe a diet based on olive oil, spaghetti and chicken is healthy. Some believe an Atkins-paleo-keto type diet with lots of meat is healthy. Some believe you can lose weight by eating the modern diet of processed food but eating less and exercising more.

There is now convincing evidence that a high-fiber, whole-food, plant-based diet of vegetables, fruit, whole grains, nuts and seeds is the optimal diet for both weight loss and good health.

According to an article on WebMD, "When it comes to losing weight, one simple piece of advice may be more helpful than all the diet books, calorie counting, and portion measuring put together: Eat more fiber."

A high-fiber diet is by definition a whole-food, plant-based diet since animal foods have no fiber and processed foods have little fiber. A high-fiber diet is a satiating (satisfying) diet that fills you up and prevents hunger between meals.

Chapters 1 and 2 review the evidence for a diet of vegetables, fruit, whole grains, nuts and seeds.

Chapter 2 on Motivation is the missing link in many diets. Diet programs often lack sustained, long-term motivational strategies. An optimal diet of the healthiest foods with quick, easy-to-prepare meals is worthless if the motivation to adopt the diet is missing. Chapter 2 provides a motivational program that conveniently and painlessly reinforces the benefits of a whole-food, plant-based diet over a period of weeks, months or years until healthy eating becomes your routine and habitual way of life.

Chapter 2 recommends audiobooks, videos and books on the benefits of a whole-food, plant-based diet. These media are widely available from libraries, bookstores and the Internet. Consuming these materials frequently and regularly provides positive reinforcement to make a healthy diet your permanent diet.

Other motivational strategies are also discussed including:

- Using a food journal to track calories and nutrients,
- Getting regular medical checkups,
- Using hypnosis or aversion therapy to associate unhealthy foods with negative images and healthy foods with positive images,

- Using online betting to gamble on weight loss,
- Joining a local TOPS club, a low-cost weight-loss support social club,
- Drinking tea or coffee to alleviate hunger between meals,
- Developing better habits with recommended books, and
- Learning National Weight Control Registry maintenance strategies.

Chapter 3 on Easy Meals describes an easy way to adopt a healthy diet. One of the reasons that processed foods and restaurants have become so popular is that they are very convenient. Healthy whole-food diet plans, on the other hand, often require a significant amount of time shopping and preparing food. Many people will not invest the time needed to follow these healthy diet recipes.

Chapter 3 provides an example of a simple, one-day meal plan that is quicker and easier to prepare than most processed food meals. Simple utensils, frozen vegetables and microwave cooking are recommended. The meals are easy and affordable to shop for, quick and easy to prepare, and quick and easy to clean up.

Chapter 4 on Exercise recommends amounts and types of aerobic and strengthening exercises.

Chapter One

Good Food

How Healthy Is Your Diet?

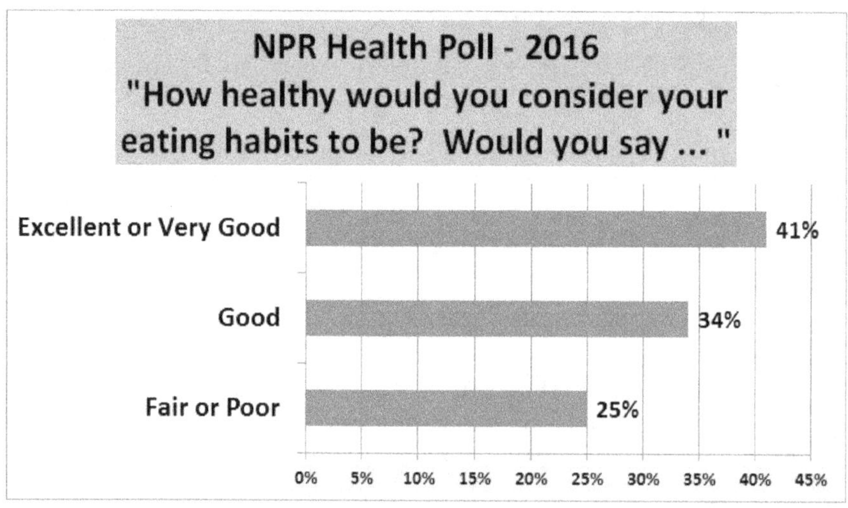

When a random sample of 3000 Americans was asked in 2016 "How healthy would you consider your eating habits to be?", 41% answered excellent or very good, 34% said good and only 25% said fair or poor.

Apparently a large majority of Americans think a diet with most calories from added fats and sugars and refined grains is a good, very good or excellent diet.

What U.S. Americans Eat

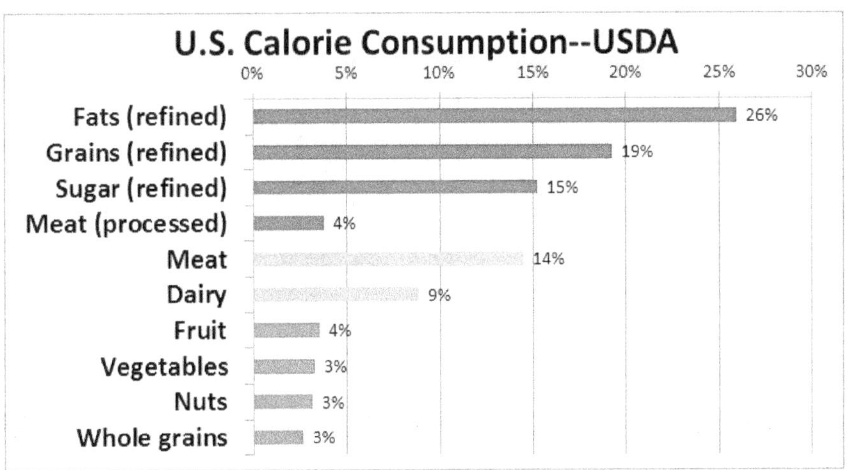

One of the jobs of the Economic Research Service of the U.S. Department of Agriculture is to keep track of calories consumed by Americans. The average American gets an amazing 60% of their calories from refined fats and oils, refined grains and refined sugars, 27% of their calories from animal foods and only 13% of calories from whole plant foods.

The chart above shows:

Four processed foods to be avoided: added fats and oils (primarily salad and cooking oils and shortening), refined grains (primarily refined wheat flour), added sugar (primarily cane and beet sugar and corn sweeteners) and processed meats (such as bacon, sausage, hot dogs and lunch meats),

Two animal foods to be eaten in moderation if at all (meat and dairy), and

Four plant foods to be eaten abundantly (fruit, vegetables, nuts and seeds and whole grains).

Refined Fats

Refined fats, what the USDA calls added fats and oils, are the leading source of calories in the modern American diet. Popular foods with added fats and oils include: French fries, fried chicken, corn and potato chips, donuts and pastries, breads, butter, bagels, rolls and biscuits, cakes, pies, muffins, cookies and salad dressings.

It's important to note that fat is not all bad. Adequate fat is essential in the human diet. The World Health Organization recommends that 15 to 30% of total calories should come from fat, 10 to 15% from protein and the balance from carbohydrates. Getting fats from nuts, seeds and avocados is a healthier, higher fiber choice than obtaining fats from deep fat fryers, baked goods and salad dressing oils.

Refined Grains

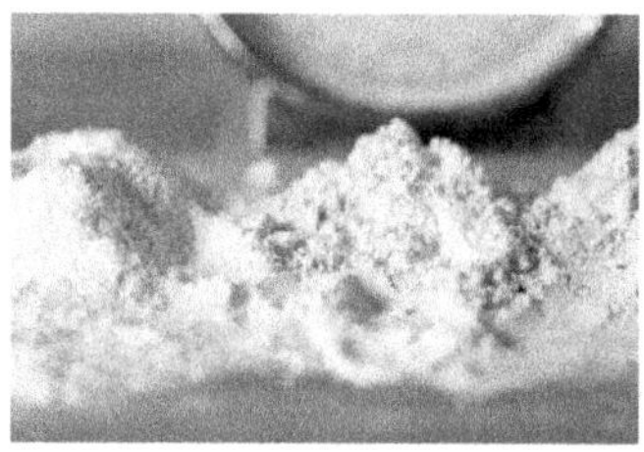

Grains, what the USDA calls flour and cereal products, are the second leading source of calories in the American diet. In 1880 the U.S. Patent Office awarded John Stevens of Wisconsin a patent for a roller milling process that allowed the germ and bran in wheat to be efficiently removed. The process made flour more affordable and extended shelf life, but also removed much of the fiber and nutrition in the wheat.

The most common American grain product by far is wheat, followed by corn and oats. Popular foods made with refined grains include: bread, dinner rolls and biscuits, pasta such as spaghetti, breakfast cereals, pizza and other mixed dishes such as hamburgers, sandwiches and tacos, cakes, cookies, pastries, donuts and muffins, white rice and other refined grains, and snack foods such as pretzels and corn chips.

Today 88% of wheat in America is refined. Only 12% is eaten whole. Removing the fiber and nutrients from grains is a serious health concern because fiber helps you feel full longer and reduces the risk of obesity, type 2 diabetes and heart disease.

A 2016 meta-analysis of 45 studies in the British Medical Journal found a significant correlation between **whole** grain consumption and a reduced risk of cardiovascular disease, cancer and all-cause mortality. There was little evidence of an association with **refined** grains or white rice. The authors recommended choosing whole grains rather than refined.

Refined Sugar

Refined sugar, what the USDA calls added sugar and sweeteners, makes up about 15% of the American diet. Nearly half of sugar calories come from sweetened beverages such as soft drinks, fruit drinks, sweetened coffee and tea, milk shakes, energy drinks and alcoholic beverages. About 30% of sugar calories come from sweets such as cakes, pies, cookies, donuts, brownies and sweet rolls, ice cream, pudding and yogurt, candies, jams, syrups, sweet toppings and table sugar. A large portion of sugar also comes from sugar added to foods such as breakfast cereals, spaghetti sauce, ketchup, salad dressing, BBQ sauce, fruit juices, canned fruit, granola bars, baked beans and crackers.

The Centers for Disease Control and Prevention says that "Americans are eating and drinking too much added sugars which can lead to health problems such as weight gain and obesity, type 2 diabetes, and heart disease." Like refined fats and oils and refined flour, refined sugar is a modern innovation that played no role in the diet of early humans.

Processed Meat

Processed meats are meats preserved by curing, salting, fermenting or smoking or the addition of chemical preservatives. 22% of meats eaten by Americans are processed meats. Examples of processed meats include: bacon, ham, beef jerky and hot dogs, salami and liverwurst, pepperoni, lunch meats, and sausages such as bratwurst. There is evidence that eating patterns that include lower intake of meats including processed meats and processed poultry are associated with reduced risk of obesity, type 2 diabetes, cardiovascular disease and some types of cancer.

Meat

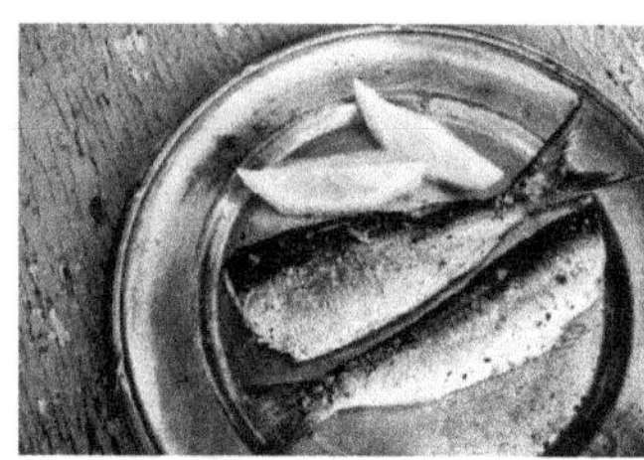

Beef and chicken in nearly equal amounts make up the majority of American meat calories with pork, eggs, turkey and fish comprising most of the remainder.

Authors like Joel Fuhrman MD, Michael Greger MD, Dean Ornish MD, Caldwell Esselstyn MD, Neal Barnard MD, T. Colin Campbell, John McDougall MD, Pamela Popper and others have argued that animal food should have a limited role or no role in a healthy diet.

Dr. Michael Greger, author of the bestseller *How Not to Die* and hundreds of short videos available at NutritionFacts.org makes a case for a meat-free diet writing: "People who eat fewer animal products have lower rates of obesity, dementia, arthritis, high blood pressure, kidney disease, gallstones, hemorrhoids, constipation, diverticulosis, and appendicitis. … Meat-free diets are even being used to reverse chronic diseases: opening clogged arteries, curing type 2 diabetes, and alleviating obesity." He goes on to say that California Adventist vegetarians "live up to 10 years longer than the average American and enjoy lower rates of heart disease, stroke, diabetes, and certain cancers."

If the goals of a healthy diet include longevity, avoidance or reversal of chronic disease and prevention or reversal of obesity, much evidence favors those who see animal foods as having at most a limited place in a healthy diet.

Autopsies of children killed in accidents show that most U.S. children have the beginnings of atherosclerotic lesions and plaques by the age of 10. Search online for "greger heart disease starts in childhood" for a short (5:50) video.

Dr. Dean Ornish, Dr. Caldwell Esselstyn and others have successfully reduced the size of atherosclerotic plaques in coronary arteries and improved blood flow with a low-fat, animal food-free diet. Coronary angiograms provide images that show their treatments work.

Since most Americans are likely to have plaque in their arteries, reversal rather than prevention should be the goal. One of the strongest arguments for limiting the role of animal food in a heart healthy diet is that atherosclerotic plaques have never been successfully treated by an animal food-based diet.

Advocates of an Atkins-paleo-keto type diet often advocate abundant consumption of meat. John McDougall MD has long advocated a whole-food, plant-based diet. He has posted a short (2:09) somewhat harsh but informative and entertaining video on YouTube titled Low Carb vs. Plant-Based comparing the authors of low carb and plant-based diets. Search online for "low carb vs plant based" in quotes. Find the 2012 version. Dr. McDougall's video makes a convincing argument that a plant-based diet is the way to achieve healthy, permanent weight loss.

Many believe that meat is needed for protein. However, plant sources provide good alternatives to meat for fats and protein. Sources of healthy fats include walnuts, almonds, ground flaxseed, chia seeds, sunflower seeds and avocados. Good sources of protein include beans, lentils, green peas, broccoli, kale and oatmeal. Plants can provide all the protein humans need.

While there is much evidence for the harmful effects of meat, there is also evidence for beneficial effects. Both a 2004 and a 2012 meta-analysis found that fish consumption may have a "beneficial effect on the prevention of CHD mortality." There may be a place for some meat in an optimal diet.

Dairy

Cheese and milk in roughly equal amounts make up the great majority of dairy products eaten by Americans with ice cream and yogurt making up a smaller portion. Most cheese is consumed as part of other dishes such as pizza, burgers, tacos and sandwiches. Most milk is consumed as a beverage or on breakfast cereals.

A study in The American Journal of Clinical Nutrition finds that "Osteoporotic bone fracture rates are highest in countries that consume the most dairy, calcium, and animal protein." There is evidence that a high-protein diet may cause calcium to be excreted in the urine. The study concludes that "Bones are better served by … increasing fruit and vegetable intakes, limiting animal protein, exercising regularly, getting adequate sunshine or supplemental vitamin D, and getting [adequate calcium] from plant sources."

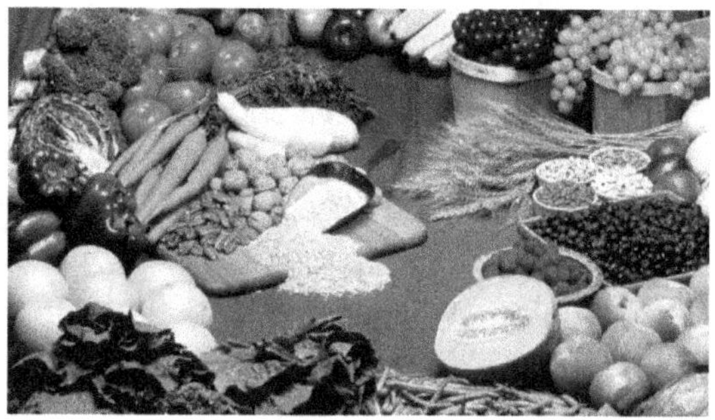

Fruit

The most popular American fruits, including 100% fruit juices, by number of calories consumed are: oranges, apples, bananas, grapes, avocados, pineapples, strawberries and pears.

A 2014 meta-analysis in the British Medical Journal of 16 studies with over 833,000 participants found that each daily serving of fruit or vegetables reduced the risk of early death by 5% up to a threshold of 5 servings. The study concluded that "higher consumption of fruit and vegetables is associated with a lower risk of all cause mortality, particularly cardiovascular mortality."

Vegetables

Examples of vegetables include: kale, tomatoes and broccoli, carrots, black and white beans and green peas, red onions, red cabbage, mushrooms and garlic.

A large meta-analysis of 95 previous studies on fruit and vegetable intake and mortality published in 2017 in the International Journal of Epidemiology found a significant correlation between fruit and vegetable intake and the prevention of cardiovascular disease, cancer and premature mortality.

Ten servings per day were found correlated with significant additional risk reduction compared to the 5 servings per day recommended by many health agencies. Apples and pears, citrus fruits, green leafy vegetables, cruciferous vegetables, and salads had the highest correlation for prevention of cardiovascular disease and all-cause mortality. Green and yellow vegetables and cruciferous vegetables had the highest correlation for reducing cancer risk.

Nuts and Seeds

Popular American nuts and seeds include: almonds, hazelnuts, pistachios and walnuts, chia seeds, ground flaxseed, pumpkin seeds and sunflower seeds. A diet that includes nuts is recommended by the American Heart Association, the Centers for Disease Control and Prevention, the U.S. Department of Agriculture and the World Health Organization.

Studies in leading nutrition journals have found that nut consumption is associated with a reduced risk of early death. One study, based on 7 prior studies, found that daily nut consumption was associated with a 27% decreased risk of all-cause mortality.

Whole Grains

Popular American whole grains include: oatmeal and bran cereals, whole grain breads and pastas, brown and wild rice and corn and popcorn. Whole grains provide much more fiber and nutrition than refined grains which have had their bran and germ removed.

According to the American Heart Association, the dietary fiber in whole grains may lower the risk of heart disease, stroke, obesity and type 2 diabetes and may help with weight loss by making you feel full.

The World Health Organization has found convincing evidence that dietary fiber reduces obesity and probable evidence that it reduces type 2 diabetes and cardiovascular disease.

A 2014 meta-analysis in the American Journal of Epidemiology found an 11% decrease in mortality for each 10 gram increase in daily dietary fiber with cereal fiber showing a stronger association than vegetable or fruit fiber.

A Healthy Diet

A plant-based diet of predominantly whole plant foods stands in sharp contrast to the modern diet of predominantly processed foods. Plant foods (vegetables, fruit, nuts, seeds and whole grains) contain fiber. Fiber slows the digestive process and provides a feeling of fullness that makes weight loss and weight maintenance much easier.

Processed foods have little or no fiber. Added fats and oils have no fiber. Added sugars have no fiber. Refined grains have little fiber. Surprisingly animal foods, both meat and dairy, have no fiber. Without adequate fiber losing weight and maintaining normal weight is difficult.

Epidemics of obesity and diabetes have followed the adoption of the modern diet of low-fiber processed foods in the United States and other countries. There is now convincing evidence that the modern diet of processed foods contributes to the prevalence of obesity, type 2 diabetes and many other chronic diseases.

Prior to the 1900s added fats and oils, refined grains and added sugars played a very minor role in the human diet. The modern diet is a radical departure from the diet of whole, unprocessed foods that humans have eaten for millions of years.

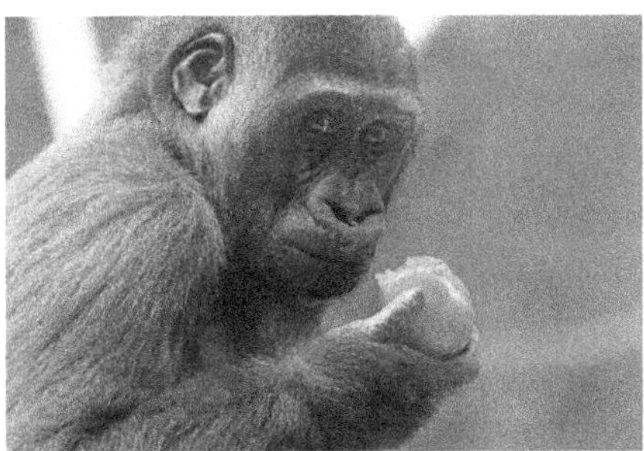

According to reference.com, "The earliest humans ate a diet similar to that of apes and chimpanzees consisting mostly of fruit and leaves ..." Refined fats, oils, grains and sugars are modern innovations that have greatly reduced the fiber and other nutrients in the human diet.

Kaiser Permanente, the largest managed care organization in the United States with over 22,000 physicians, in its 20-page booklet "The Plant-Based Diet: A Healthy Way to Eat" writes that a "low-fat, whole foods, plant-based diet ... includes lots of plant foods in their whole, unprocessed form, such as vegetables, fruits, beans, lentils, nuts, seeds, whole grains, and small amounts of healthy fats. It does not include animal products, such as meat, poultry, fish, dairy, and eggs. It also does not include processed foods or sweets."

The booklet lists some of "the benefits of a plant-based diet" including "lower cholesterol, blood pressure, and blood sugar, reversal or prevention of heart disease, longer life, healthier weight, lower risk of cancer and diabetes, may slow the progression of certain types of cancer, improved symptoms of rheumatoid arthritis, fewer medications, lower food costs, good for the environment".

T. Colin Campbell in his 2014 book *The Low-Carb Fraud* summarizes the optimal human diet: "Good science tells us the optimal way to eat is what I call the Whole-food, Plant-Based (WFPB) diet. ... The WFPB diet consists of whole foods—that is, foods as close to their natural state as possible. A wide variety of fruits, vegetables, grains, nuts, and seeds make up the bulk of the diet. It includes no refined products, such as white sugar or white flour; no additives, preservatives, or other chemical concoctions, which our bodies were never programmed to recognize or digest; no refined fats, including olive or coconut oils; and minimal—or, better yet, no—consumption of animal products, perhaps 0 to 5 percent of total calories at most."

The **World Health Organization** and the United Nations in a 2002 report titled *Human Vitamin and Mineral Requirements*, after years of consultation by leading nutrition scientists from around the world, recommended a diet "based primarily on foods of plant origin with small amounts of added flesh foods. Households should select predominantly plant-based diets rich in a variety of vegetables and fruits, pulses or legumes, and minimally processed starchy staple foods. The evidence that such diets will prevent or delay a significant proportion of non-communicable chronic diseases is consistent. A predominantly plant-based diet has a low energy density, which may protect against obesity."

The World Health Organization in its 2003 report, *Diet, Nutrition and the Prevention of Chronic Diseases*, page 56, recommends the following proportion of macronutrients:

- Protein 10-15%,
- Fat 15-30%
- Carbohydrates 55-75%

Cronometer.com, a free online food journal, shows the proportions of macronutrients in a diet.

The November 2005 edition of **National Geographic** published a cover story titled "The Secrets of Long Life" about the centenarians of Okinawa, Japan, Sardinia, Italy and Loma Linda, California. One of the secrets is a plant-based diet of whole foods. The article mentions "Chinese radishes, garlic, scallions, cabbage, turmeric, and tomatoes" for Okinawans, "zucchini, eggplant, tomatoes, and fava beans" for Sardinians, and oatmeal, nuts, beans and tomatoes for Adventists. Search online for "greger okinawa diet" for a short (5:05) video by Dr. Michael Greger on the Okinawan and Adventist diets.

A Satisfying, High-Fiber Diet

One reason that diets fail is that most people go about dieting all wrong. If you try to follow the standard advice to "eat less and exercise more" and continue eating the standard modern diet of processed foods, you are very likely to be part of the majority of diets that fail. Processed foods are deficient in fiber and nutrients. Only whole plant foods provide the bulk, fiber and nutrients needed for healthy, long-term weight loss.

The key to successful weight loss is eating high-fiber foods and avoiding processed foods. To lose weight eat whole foods and eliminate processed foods from your kitchen and your diet.

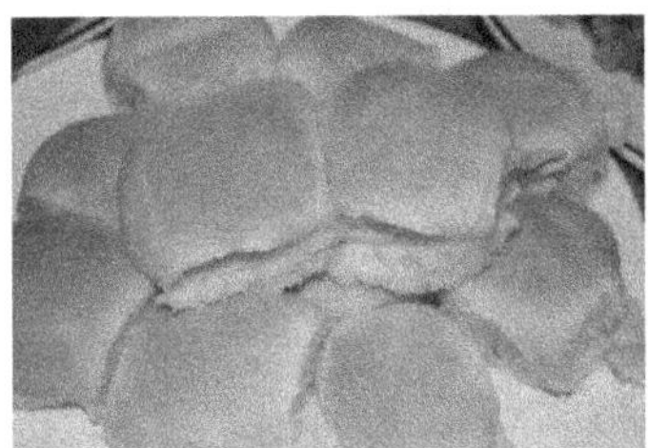

The modern diet is made up predominantly of processed foods. Major types of processed foods include:

- Breads, pastas, breakfast cereals, crackers and other foods made of refined flour,
- Cakes, cookies, candy, ice cream and other sweets,
- Soda pop, fruit juices and other sweetened beverages, and
- Sausages, hot dogs, salami, bacon, ham and other processed meats.

An article in **Food Today** "What makes us feel full? The satiating power of foods" describes the process by which foods create a feeling of fullness: "During a meal, the stomach expands, and internal nerve receptors sense the volume of food and the pressure on the stomach wall. These receptors send signals to the brain via the vagus nerve, causing the sensation of fullness. ... Fruit and vegetables-especially boiled potatoes-proved to have high satiating values, whereas bakery products like cakes, croissants and biscuits were the least satiating foods."

Satisfying, satiating foods that prevent hunger between meals have two important characteristics:

- They have a high water content, and
- They have a high fiber content.

Foods with water and fiber provide bulk that makes us feel full, but the fiber in the foods add few calories and the water adds no calories. Whole plant foods are often high in water and fiber and high in nutrients, making them ideal foods for both weight loss and good health. Processed foods usually have little fiber, little water and few nutrients.

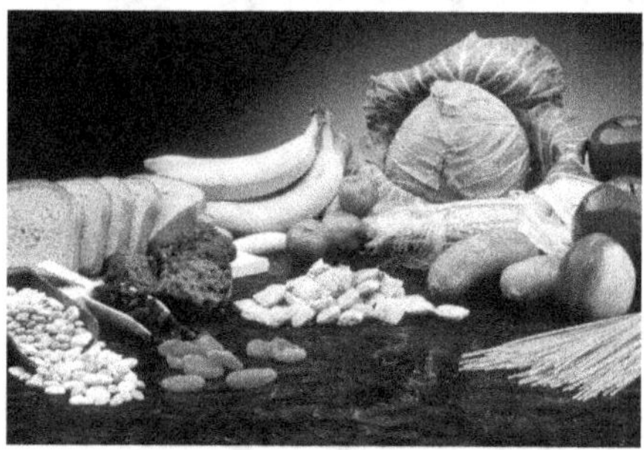

Leading dietary authorities support the importance of fiber and the need to eat foods with low calorie density (i.e., low in calories for their weight) such as fruits and vegetables for successful weight loss:

The **World Health Organization** in a 2003 report titled *"Diet, Nutrition and the Prevention of Chronic Diseases"* (p. 63) found convincing evidence that high-fiber foods "such as fruit, legumes, vegetables and whole grain cereals" prevented weight gain and obesity and that "processed foods that are high in fat and/or sugars" promoted weight gain and obesity.

The **USDA** in a report titled "Dietary Energy Density and Body Weight: A Review of the Evidence" reviewed major studies on the relationship between energy density (ED) and weight loss/weight maintenance. The report concluded that there was "strong and consistent evidence in adults that dietary patterns that are relatively low in ED [energy density] improve weight loss and weight maintenance." The report concluded:

"The Dietary Guidelines for Americans, 2010 encourages consumption of an eating pattern low in ED. An eating pattern low in ED is characterized by a relatively high intake of vegetables, fruit, and dietary fiber and a relatively low intake of total fat, saturated fat, and added sugars. The 2010 DGA noted that consuming an eating pattern low in ED may help to reduce calorie intake and improve body weight outcomes. The 2010 DGA also noted that eating patterns low in ED may be associated with improved overall health, including a lower risk of type 2 diabetes in adults."

The American Heart Association, in an article titled "Fiber Up, Slim Down" on its website, concurs with the USDA on the importance of a high-fiber diet for weight loss:

"Losing weight can be a frustrating experience if you feel hungry all the time. Did you know you can curb your appetite — and your frustration with weight-loss efforts — by increasing the amount of fiber you eat?

High-fiber foods may help you lose weight by helping you feel full on fewer calories. A healthy diet of lower-calorie foods and regular physical activity is your best strategy for achieving a healthy weight – and maintaining it. ...

High-fiber foods often require more chewing and may take longer for your stomach to digest. This can help your body recognize that it is full, before you start eating more food. Diets rich in whole grains and fiber have been associated with better quality diets and decreased risk of cardiovascular disease."

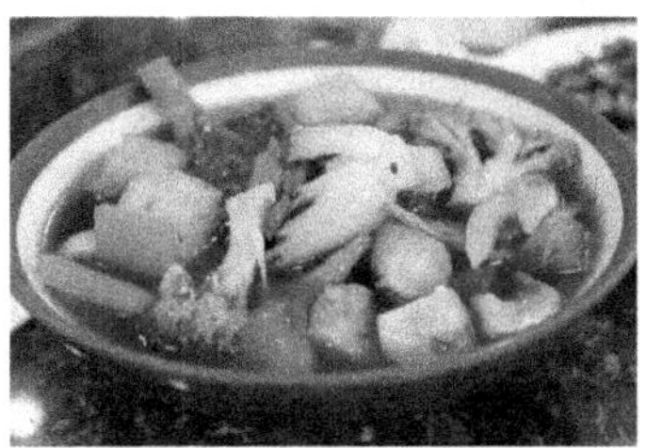

The **CDC** (Centers for Disease Control and Prevention) in a research review titled "Can eating fruits and vegetables help people to manage their weight?" concluded that:

"[R]eplacing foods of high energy density (high calories per weight of food) with foods of lower energy density, such as fruits and vegetables, can be an important part of a weight management strategy. ...

People may not limit what they consume based on calories alone. Feeling full is one reason that people stop eating. Short-term studies indicate that the volume of food people eat at a meal is what makes them feel full and stop eating, rather than the calorie content of the food."

Until you learn how to reduce and prevent hunger, weight loss and long-term weight maintenance will be difficult. In a pamphlet titled "Eat More, Weigh Less? How to manage your weight without being hungry", the CDC says:

"Have you tried to lose weight by cutting down the amount of food you eat? Do you end up feeling hungry and not satisfied? ... You can cut calories without eating less nutritious food. The key is to eat foods that will fill you up without eating a large amount of calories. ... Research shows that people get full by the amount of food they eat, not the number of calories they take in. ... Foods that have a lot of water and fiber and little fat are usually low in calorie density. They will help you feel full without an unnecessary amount of calories."

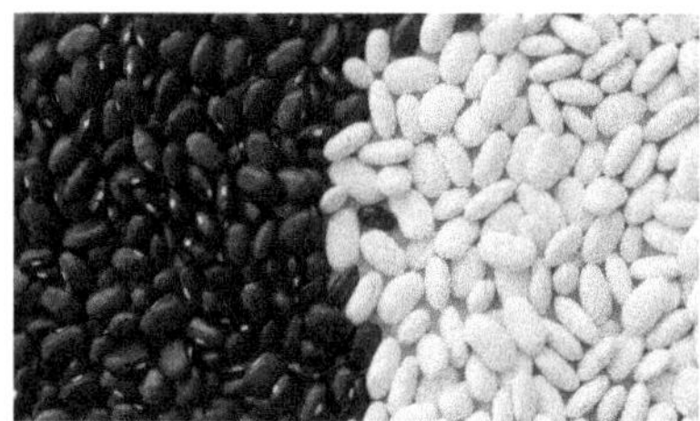

The **Academy of Nutrition and Dietetics**, the largest organization of food and nutrition professionals in the United States, agrees on the importance of fiber. Their advice:

"Focus on the big picture—achieving overall good health—not just short-term weight loss. ... Get plenty of fiber from fruits, vegetables, beans and whole grains. Fiber can help you feel full longer and lower your risk for heart disease and type 2 diabetes."

An article on **WebMD** titled "High-Fiber Diets and Weight Loss" summarizes the case for fiber:

"When it comes to losing weight, one simple piece of advice may be more helpful than all the diet books, calorie counting, and portion measuring put together: Eat more fiber.

A recent study ... added to a growing body of evidence that people who eat more fiber tend to have a healthier body weight.

While high-fiber foods tend to be healthy (think: fruit, veggies, whole grains), what proved equally important was that this kind of diet was easier to stick to...

How exactly does fiber guard against hunger pangs? Simple: It fills your stomach, stimulating receptors that tell your brain that it's time to stop eating."

Barbara Rolls PhD co-authored *The Ultimate Volumetrics Diet: Smart, Simple, Science-Based Strategies for Losing Weight and Keeping It Off* (HarperCollins, 2012) on the importance of fiber and calorie density for weight loss.

Dr. Dean Ornish wrote *Eat More, Weigh Less* (Harper Collins, 1993). Dr. Ornish shows that by eating the right foods, you can eat abundantly and lose weight. Low-calorie, high-fiber, high-nutrient foods are a key ingredient of a healthy diet and of a sustainable, long-term weight maintenance eating plan.

Dr. Greger has a short (5:06) video on what ancient humans may have eaten and the importance of fiber in combating obesity. There is evidence that the earliest humans may have consumed 100 grams (about 3.5 ounces) or more of fiber a day. Modern humans who rely on processed foods often eat less than 20 grams of fiber a day. Search online for "greger paleopoo" for the video.

Healthy eating is not so much about willpower and eating less. It's about eating the right, satisfying, high-nutrient, high-fiber, high-water-content and usually low-calorie foods that allow you to eat enough to satiate your hunger.

Unlike the modern, processed-food, low-fiber diet, a healthy, plant-based diet is high in fiber and very satiating. To avoid problems with excessive fiber, be sure to drink plenty of water and other fluids on a high-fiber diet.

Fasting

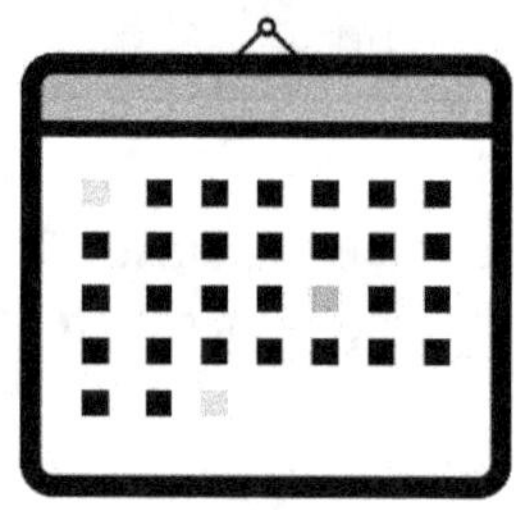

A strategy that may be effective for people who hit a weight loss plateau and for long-term weight loss maintenance is intermittent fasting.

One popular method is the 5:2 diet in which a single meal of about 500 calories is eaten on two non-consecutive days each week and regular meals the other days.

A 2015 article in the International Journal of Obesity (Johnstone, Fasting for weight loss: an effective strategy or latest dieting trend?) concluded that "Intermittent fasting or alternate day fasting may be an option for achieving weight loss and maintenance."

An online article by Authority Nutrition (Kris Gunnars, Intermittent Fasting 101 – The Ultimate Beginner's Guide) explains some of the methods, benefits and risks of intermittent fasting.

Benefits of fasting that are cited include improved insulin sensitivity and cellular repair. Also fasting may simplify your life by reducing the number of meals you need to prepare.

The article points out that while intermittent fasting may be an effective weight loss tool for many, it is not for everyone.

Dr. Joel Fuhrman is the author of a 1995 book on fasting titled *Fasting and Eating for Health: A Medical Doctor's Program for Conquering Disease.* Dr. Neal Barnard wrote the Foreword.

The Amazon review says the book "offers precise diet and fasting programs to relieve headache, hypoglycemia, rheumatoid arthritis, asthma, heart disease, high blood pressure, diabetes, colitis, psoriasis, lupus, and uterine fibroids. You'll also learn: How to use fasting to lose weight …"

Dr. Michael Greger has published several videos on caloric restriction on his NutritionFacts.org website:

- Is caloric restriction good for you?
- Why do we age?
- Caloric restriction vs. animal protein restriction
- Caloric restriction vs. plant-based diets
- The Okinawa diet: living to 100

Dr. Alan Goldhamer with Dr. John McDougall has produced a long (1 hour, 25 minute) online video titled "Fasting: an ancient practice for modern problems".

Dr. Dean Ornish has endorsed intermittent fasting in a Twitter post: "Occasional fasting is good for your health, if done properly. If you can fast one day a week, or one day a month, or one day every few..."

Chapter Two

Motivation

Changing Habits

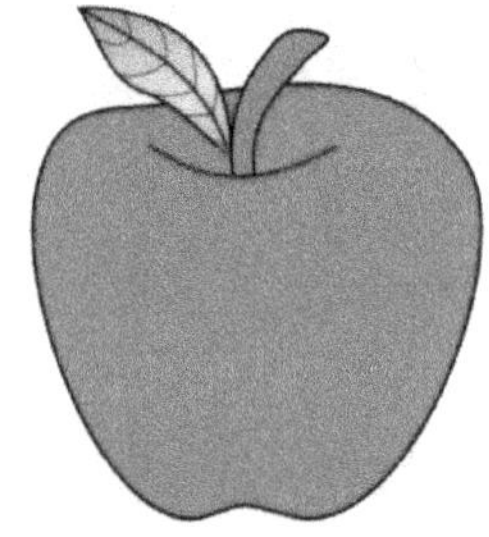

The threads of habit are too light to be felt until they're too strong to be broken. This is true of both good habits and bad habits. Feelings and thoughts about food are formed gradually over many years beginning in childhood. Long-ingrained habits cannot be changed instantly in a sudden burst of enthusiasm.

Changing eating habits that have developed over many years begins with learning about the benefits of a healthy diet. This is a gradual process of education that takes time to accomplish.

Fortunately there is a rich literature of entertaining books, articles, audiobooks and videos on the benefits of a whole-food, plant-based diet. This chapter lists and describe some of these resources.

The recommended audiobooks, videos and books provide convincing evidence of the benefits of a healthy, high-fiber diet. However there are strong forces in modern society promoting low-fiber, processed foods and making these foods very convenient and appealing.

A sustained, documented program of listening, watching and reading is necessary to change long-ingrained eating habits. *Our thoughts make our habits, then our habits make us.*

Habits take time to form and time to replace. Bad eating habits may take weeks of listening to audiobooks, watching videos and daily reading to replace with healthy eating habits.

Education on the benefits of a healthy diet requires an investment of time. However it's a very effective way to change habits and behavior. According to American psychologist B.F. Skinner, "Properly used, positive reinforcement is extremely powerful".

Keep a daily record of audiobooks you listen to, videos you watch and materials you read. Keep up this program of education and daily record keeping for several weeks or several months until eating whole foods is your routine and habitual way of eating.

Listen and relisten to the recommended audiobooks, watch and rewatch the videos, immerse yourself in the books until a healthy diet becomes automatic and routine. If you do this and keep a simple daily record you'll be well on your way to adopting a healthy diet.

Focus on material that advocates a healthy, plant-based diet. Don't be distracted by diets that advocate excessive consumption of animal foods. As discussed in the previous chapter, the idea that animal foods are needed for adequate protein is a myth that is not supported by the evidence.

Spend as much time as possible listening to audiobooks and watching videos with members of your household with whom you share meals. It's easier to adopt a healthy diet if members of your household share the same diet.

Continue learning about the advantages of a healthy diet. After a healthy diet is firmly established, the benefits of a whole-food, plant-based diet should be regularly reinforced with a long-term program of audiobooks, videos and reading.

Getting Started

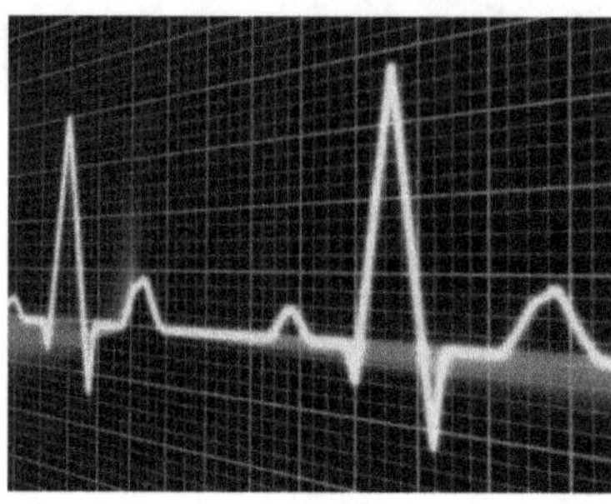

Start by reading the publication you're reading right now. As you read, follow the links to videos and watch those videos. *Get Healthy* is an effective way to adopt a healthy diet.

Consider British author and preacher Charles Spurgeon's advice on books: "Peruse a good book several times and make notes and analyses of it. A student will find that his mental constitution is more affected by one book thoroughly mastered than by twenty books he has merely skimmed."

Next get a copy of *Eat to Live* by Joel Fuhrman MD. *Eat to Live* is not perfect. Dr. Fuhrman's views on coffee may be out-of-date. His recipes and meal plans are often too time-consuming and inconvenient for busy people who don't want to spend much time in the kitchen on food preparation and clean-up.

Nevertheless *Eat to Live* is an amazing book that has helped countless people (including myself many years ago) to adopt and follow a whole-food, plant-based diet. The book makes a convincing case that a "nutritarian" diet is the best way to lose weight and to prevent and reverse heart disease, type 2 diabetes and many other chronic diseases. Copies of *Eat to Live* are inexpensive on Amazon and widely available at libraries.

Two of Dr. Fuhrman's other books, *The End of Heart Disease*, and *The End of Diabetes* (available in both book and audiobook format) are also recommended.

Another amazing author to start reading and listening to is Michael Greger MD. Dr. Greger is the author of the runaway bestseller *How Not to Die: Discover the Foods Scientifically Proven to Prevent and Reverse Disease*. He is also the author of *How Not to Diet: The*

Groundbreaking Science of Permanent Weight Loss. Both of these books are available in both book and audiobook format.

Dr. Greger is also the author and narrator of over two thousand videos that are freely available at NutritionFacts.org. Search online for "greger why you should care about nutrition" for a short (2:53) video on the importance of a healthy diet for reducing the risks of disability and death.

Two other resources that provide a good overview of the leading authors and benefits of a whole-food, plant-based diet are: *The Whole Foods Diet* (John Mackey et al) and a video by Plant Based News (13:23) "shocking effects of a whole food plant based vegan diet".

Audiobooks

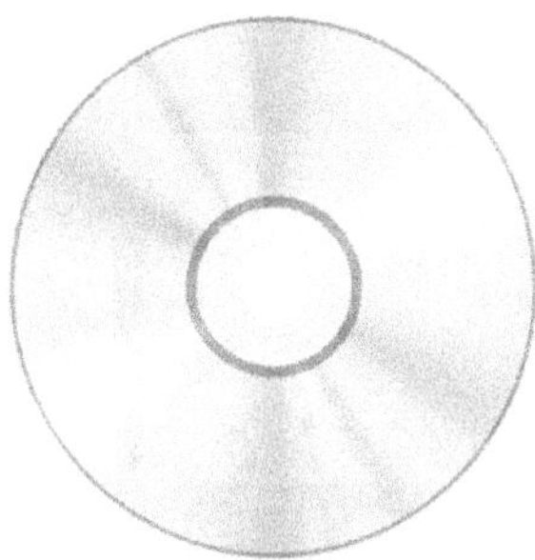

Audiobooks are great. They make it easy to learn about and to reinforce the benefits of a whole-food, plant-based diet. Get a CD player or other type of audio player to keep by your bed at night. Listen to audiobooks as you go to sleep and if you wake up at night.

Listen to audiobooks as you drive. Listen as you walk or exercise. Advertising research has found that a message may need to be heard many times before it is effective at changing behavior. Listen to these audiobooks repeatedly until eating a healthy diet becomes routine.

Check local libraries, regional libraries and stores for the following audiobooks which are available in both book and audiobook format:

- *Eat to Live*, Joel Fuhrman MD
- *How Not to Die*, Michael Greger MD
- *How Not to Diet*, Michael Greger MD
- *The China Study* (2016 edition), T. Colin Campbell and

Thomas M. Campbell MD

- *The End of Heart Disease*, Joel Fuhrman MD
- *The End of Dieting*, Joel Fuhrman MD
- *The End of Diabetes*, Joel Fuhrman MD
- *Disease-Proof Your Child*, Joel Fuhrman MD
- *Eat for Health*, Joel Fuhrman MD
- *Dr. Neal Barnard's Program for Reversing Diabetes*, Neal Barnard MD
- *The Low-Carb Fraud*, T. Colin Campbell
- *Whole*, T. Colin Campbell and Howard Jacobsen
- *The Spectrum*, Dean Ornish MD.

Videos

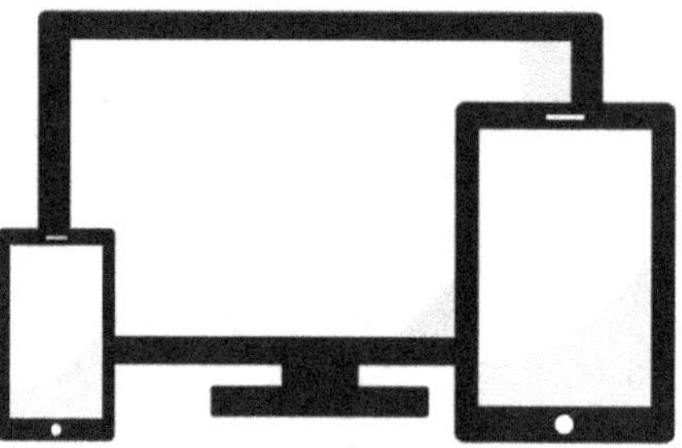

A sustained program of learning with videos is an easy and effective way to adopt and follow a healthy diet.

Online videos: Internet sites such as NutritionFacts.org and YouTube are sources of free videos.

NutritionFacts.org by Michael Greger MD:

- *Taking Personal Responsibility for Your Health* (3:58)
- *The Story of Nutrition Facts.org* (3:17)
- *Why You Should Care About Nutrition* (2:54)
- *How Not to Die: Preventing, Arresting, and Reversing Our Top 15 Killers* (82 min)
- *Food as Medicine: Preventing and Treating the Most Dreaded Diseases with Diet* (75 min)
- *From Table to Able: Combating Disabling Diseases with Food* (54

min)
- *More Than an Apple a Day: Preventing the Most Common Diseases* (62 min)
- *Uprooting the Leading Causes of Death* (56 min)
- *Evidence-Based Weight Loss: Live Presentation* (60 min)

From NutritionFacts.org, click Video Library, then Browse Videos by Topic for a list of hundreds of short videos. Subscribe to receive videos by email.

Search **YouTube** for leading advocates of a healthy, plant-based diet:
- Joel Fuhrman
- Michael Greger
- Neal Barnard
- Dean Ornish
- Caldwell Esselstyn
- Colin Campbell
- Pamela Popper
- Michael Klaper
- John McDougall

Search online for "free mcdougall program" for Dr. McDougall's free online program.

DVD videos: You may have access to these videos through your local library:
- *Processed People: The Documentary* (2009, 205 min)
- *The Weight of the Nation* (2012, 276 min)
- *Forks Over Knives* (2011, 96 min)
- *Planeat* (2011, 72 min)
- *Chow Down* (2010, 73 min)
- *Eating for Cancer Survival* (Neal Barnard, 2009, 270 min)

Search for other DVDs using the names of authors who advocate a whole-food, plant-based diet.

Get Healthy Now! VegSource.com has held conferences on plant-based nutrition since the early 2000s. There is a 3-DVD set (approx.13 hours each) for 11 of the conferences from 2005 to 2016. Amazon describes the 2015 video set as "13 hours of inspiring, enlightening, life-saving information!" These videos are available for sale from VegSource.com and from some public libraries.

Devote time on a regular, long-term basis to watching videos until healthy eating is normal and habitual.

Books

In addition to the books listed above that are available in both book and audiobook format, the following are recommended:

- *The Whole Foods Diet,* John Mackey et al
- *Prevent and Reverse Heart Disease*, Caldwell Esselstyn, Jr. MD
- *21-Day Weight Loss Kickstart*, Neal Barnard MD
- *The Good Carbohydrate Revolution*, Terry Shintani MD, JD
- *Food over Medicine: The Conversation That Could Save Your Life*, Pamela Popper
- *The Full Plate Diet*, Stuart Seale MD et al
- *The Mayo Clinic Diet, 2nd Edition*, Donald Hensrud MD
- *The Starch Solution*, John McDougall MD
- *The Healthiest Diet on the Planet*, John McDougall MD

Other Strategies

A long-sustained program of listening to audiobooks, watching videos and reading books on the benefits of a healthy diet is an effective strategy for adopting and following a new way of eating. However there may be strong forces at work pushing you to continue eating a diet of processed foods.

Often the main obstacle is people you live and eat with who don't embrace your new diet. It's important to persuade your spouse or other household members of the benefits of a plant-based diet. As mentioned previously listening to audiobooks and watching videos together is one way to do this. It may take patience and persistence and additional motivational strategies to strengthen your resolve and convince your household to work with you on adopting a healthy diet.

Fortunately there are other effective motivational strategies. In addition to a program of listening, watching videos and reading to reinforce the benefits of a healthy diet, these additional tools are recommended.

A Food Journal

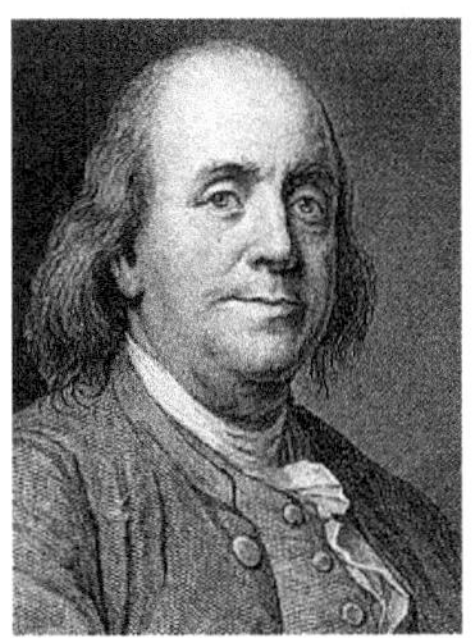

Benjamin Franklin in his *Autobiography* writes of his "plan for attaining moral perfection" by focusing on one of 13 virtues each week and keeping a record with a mark in his daily log of his failures to apply that virtue. In a similar way a daily food journal focuses attention on following a healthy diet. It's often easier to pass on eating some unhealthy food than having to account for it on a daily food log.

The Cronometer food journal at cronometer.com has a free and a paid version and a large database of foods for tracking daily calories and nutrients. Cronometer allows you to see what nutrients may be deficient or excessive in your diet. By allowing copying and pasting from a previous day the food journal can be completed quickly each day.

Medical Checkups

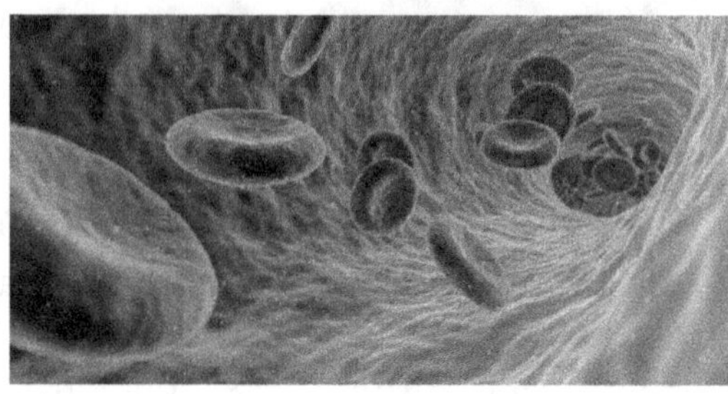

Know your medical numbers such as weight, waistline, blood lipids (cholesterol, triglycerides), blood glucose (A1c), and blood pressure. Tracking your medical numbers provides information about your health and incentive to improve.

Blood pressure, blood glucose and cholesterol may improve rapidly on a whole-food, plant-based diet. Search online for "ncbi effect of a high nutrient density diet" for the abstract of one study. When you see improvement in your numbers, you'll have additional motivation to follow a healthy, plant-based diet.

For a booklet describing the preventive medical tests that Medicare provides at no charge to eligible patients, search online for "your guide to Medicare preventive services". For example, many on Medicare are eligible for diabetes screenings to determine their A1c number. A1c measures your average blood glucose level over the last 3 months. This number tells you if you are diabetic or pre-diabetic and provides incentive to lower your A1c number by improving your diet and avoiding high-fat and sugary foods.

Hypnosis and Aversion

Hypnosis is a state of relaxed meditation characterized by heightened susceptibility to suggestion. It has been used successfully to change many behaviors including smoking, alcoholism, overeating and nail biting. Many studies have been done on the effectiveness of hypnosis for weight loss.

A 1985 study (Bolocofsky et al, Effectiveness of hypnosis as an adjunct to behavioral weight management) of 109 subjects found that the addition of hypnosis to a weight loss program resulted in significant additional weight loss at the 8-month and 2-year follow-ups.

A 1986 study (Cochrane, Hypnotherapy in weight loss treatment) divided 60 women into 2 groups. One group got weight loss counseling. The other got weight loss counseling plus hypnosis. At the end of 6 months the counseling only group lost an average of ½ pound. The counseling plus hypnosis group lost an average of 17 pounds.

A 1996 meta-analysis (Kirsch, Hypnotic enhancement of cognitive-behavioral weight loss treatments) found that average weight loss was 6.03 pounds without hypnosis and 14.88 pounds with hypnosis.

Aversion therapy is a type of hypnotic suggestion in which a food you wish to avoid is associated with negative images. For example you might imagine a food you want to avoid as infested with maggots, worms or ants. This can be an effective strategy. A YouTube video by Joseph Kuhn MD titled "Aversion hypnosis therapy for food addiction" provides an example of aversion therapy.

DietBet.com

DietBet.com is a website that uses competition to promote weight loss and weight loss maintenance. Participants choose from 3 games: (1) a kickstarter 'lose a little' game that lasts 4 weeks and aims to lose 4% of body weight; (2) a transformer 'lose a lot' game that lasts 6 months and aims to lose 10% of body weight; and (3) a maintainer 'hold steady' game that lasts 12 months and aims to maintain body weight within +2%. Participants pay to play with successful players sharing the pot after payment of DietBet's fee of up to 25%.

According to DietBet, "Players have lost 5 million pounds and we've paid out over $21 million to winners. Dietbetting is now a worldwide movement with over 400,000 players in 90 countries."

TOPS Club

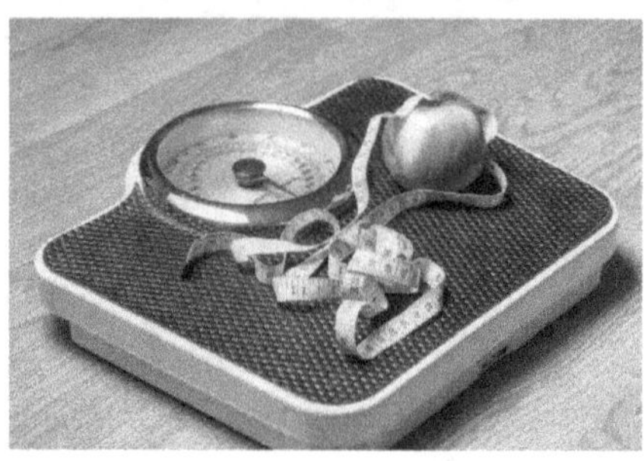

TOPS Club, Inc. is a non-profit corporation that organizes support groups for people trying to lose weight and maintain weight loss. Founded in 1948, TOPS is an acronym for Take Off Pounds Sensibly. TOPS has 180,000 members and 10,000 chapters located throughout the world but primarily in the United States and Canada. There are many active chapters. For example, in the Denver area within 10 miles of 80210 there are 14 chapters.

Each chapter holds a weekly weigh-in followed by a meeting. A meeting might include a group recitation of affirmations, a financial report, a report of successful "losers" who may be entitled to a one dollar prize, a report of total weight lost for the year by all the chapter members collectively, a short statement by each member of high and low points of their week, a book report by a member that might discuss food, health, exercise or motivation, and recitation of a closing affirmation with everyone holding hands around the table. After the half-hour weigh-in period, the meeting lasts about an hour.

Members who reach their weight goal (set by their healthcare provider) are recognized as KOPS (Keep Off Pounds Sensibly). At the time of this writing, there is an annual membership fee of $32 in the United States ($36 in Canada) plus weekly dues of a dollar or two to pay for prizes to successful "losers".

Coffee and Tea

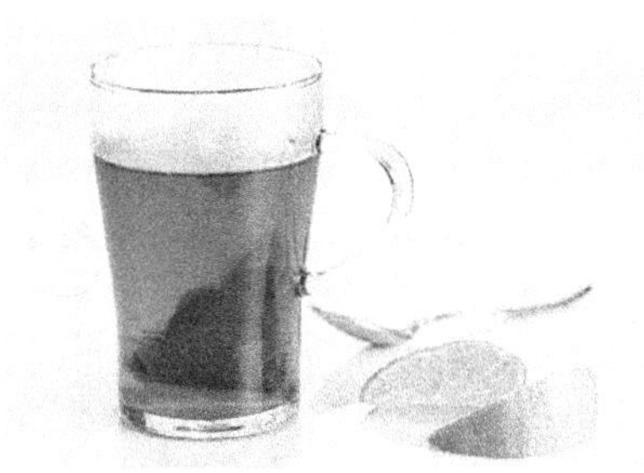

If you feel hungry between meals, is there anything you can eat or drink to satisfy your hunger?

A 2010 study (Josic et al, Does green tea affect postprandial glucose, insulin and satiety in healthy subjects: a randomized controlled trial) concluded that "Green tea showed no glucose or insulin-lowering effect. However, increased satiety and fullness were reported by the participants after the consumption of green tea."

A 2012 study (Greenberg et al, Coffee, hunger, and peptide YY) found that coffee could decrease hunger and increase satiety. There is increasing evidence that coffee may not be the unhealthy drink it was once thought to be. Even the National Cancer Institute reported recently on a study which found that coffee drinkers "were less likely to die from heart disease, respiratory disease, stroke, injuries and accidents, diabetes and infections".

Habit Strategies

Find strategies that work for you to break bad habits and establish good habits by reading and listening to audiobooks.

Two recommended books (also available as audiobooks):

(1) *Atomic Habits: Tiny changes, remarkable results: an easy & proven way to build good habits & break bad ones,* James Clear (2018 & 2019)

(2) *The 7 Habits of Highly Effective People: Powerful lessons in personal change,* Stephen R. Covey (2013)

Use the books and audiobooks above to form the habit of using audiobooks, videos and books each day until a healthy diet becomes your routine way of eating.

National Weight Control Registry

The National Weight Control Registry (NWCR), founded by Rena Wing and James Hill in 1994, is an ongoing, long-term research study of people who have lost a significant amount of weight and have succeeded at keeping the weight off. The average adult who has joined the study had lost about 66 pounds and kept the weight off for over 5 years. Over 10,000 members have joined over the years making it the largest prospective study of long-term weight maintenance. Current members complete a detailed questionnaire each year that asks about weight, health, diet, exercise, lifestyle choices such as television-watching and self-weighing, and other motivational strategies for keeping weight off long term.

A 2005 study by one of the co-founders of the NWCR (Wing et al, Long-term weight loss maintenance) reported successful strategies used by members: "To maintain their weight loss, members report engaging in high levels of physical activity (approximately 1 h/d), eating a low-calorie, low-fat diet, eating breakfast regularly, self-monitoring weight, and maintaining a consistent eating pattern across weekdays and weekends. Moreover, weight loss maintenance may get easier over time; after individuals have successfully maintained their weight loss for 2-5 y, the chance of longer-term success greatly increases. Continued adherence to diet and exercise strategies, low levels of depression and disinhibition [loss of self-control], and medical triggers for weight loss are also associated with long-term success. National Weight Control Registry members provide evidence that long-term weight loss maintenance is possible and help identify the specific approaches associated with long-term success."

A 2005 study by the other co-founder of the NWCR (Hill et al, The National Weight Control Registry: is it useful in helping deal with our obesity epidemic?) also reported on successful weight loss maintenance strategies: "To maintain their weight loss NWCR participants report eating a relatively low-fat diet, eating breakfast almost every day, weighing themselves regularly, and engaging in high levels (about 1 hour/day) of physical activity. … The value of this project lies in identifying potential strategies that may help others be more successful in keeping weight off."

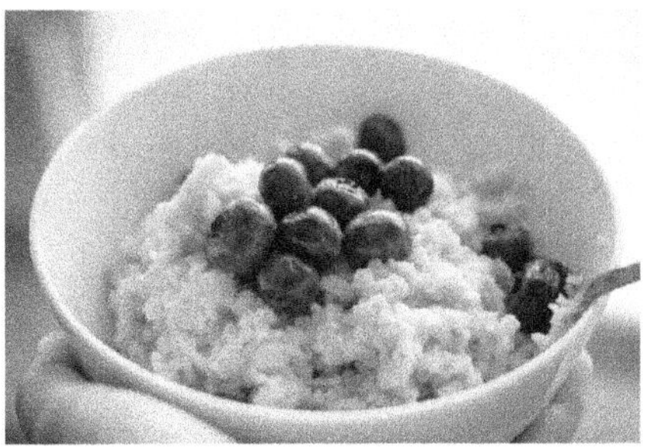

Eat breakfast

A 2002 study (Wyatt et al, Long-term weight loss and breakfast in subjects in the National Weight Control Registry) focuses on eating breakfast. "A large proportion of NWCR subjects (2313 or 78%) reported regularly eating breakfast every day of the week. … Eating breakfast is a characteristic common to successful weight loss maintainers and may be a factor in their success."

Eat an unvarying diet

Two studies have focused on the importance of eating a consistent diet for weight loss maintenance even if the variety of foods eaten is limited. A 2004 study (Gorin et al, Promoting long-term weight control: does dieting consistency matter?) reported: "The present study examined whether long-term weight loss maintenance is enhanced by maintaining the same diet regimen across the week and year or by dieting more strictly on weekdays and nonholiday periods than at other times. … Participants who reported a consistent diet across the week were 1.5 times more likely to maintain their weight within 5 pounds over the subsequent year … Dieting consistency appears to be a behavioral strategy that predicts subsequent long-term weight loss maintenance."

A 2005 study (Raynor et al, Amount of food group variety consumed in the diet and long-term weight loss maintenance) reported similar findings: "At entry into the registry, registry members completed a food frequency questionnaire from which amount of variety consumed from different food groups was assessed. … Registry members reported consuming a diet with very low variety in all food groups, especially in those food groups higher in fat density. ... These results suggest that successful weight loss maintainers consume a diet with limited variety in all food groups. Restricting variety within all food groups may help with consuming a low-energy diet and maintaining long-term weight loss."

Exercise

A 2007 study (Phelan et al, Empirical evaluation of physical activity recommendations for weight control in women) on the duration and intensity of exercise needed to maintain weight loss reports: "Recent recommendations advise 30-60 min of physical activity per day to prevent weight gain and 60-90 min to prevent weight regain. ... Findings support current recommendations that more activity may be needed to prevent weight regain than to prevent weight gain. Including some higher-intensity activity may also be advisable for weight-loss maintenance."

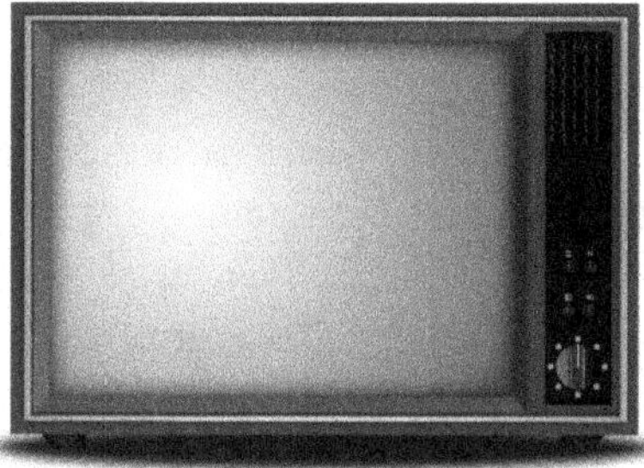

Watch less TV

A 2006 study (Raynor et al, Television viewing and long-term weight maintenance: results from the National Weight Control Registry) examines the role of television viewing on long-term weight loss maintenance: "A relatively high proportion (62.3%) of participants reported watching 10 or fewer hours of TV per week on entry in the NWCR. More than one third of the sample (36.1%) reported watching <5 h/wk, whereas only 12.4% watched > or =21 h/wk, which contrasts markedly from the national average of 28 hours of TV viewing per week reported by American adults. ...

Individuals who are successful at maintaining weight loss over the long term are likely to spend a relatively minimal amount of time watching TV."

Weigh yourself often

A 2007 study (Butryn et al, Consistent self-monitoring of weight: a key component of successful weight loss maintenance) recommends frequent self-weighing to maintain weight loss: "Consistent self-weighing may help individuals maintain their successful weight loss by allowing them to catch weight gains before they escalate and make behavior changes to prevent additional weight gain."

Medical events trigger weight loss

A 2004 study (Gorin et al, Medical triggers are associated with better short- and long-term weight loss outcomes) found that adverse medical events are often the motivation for weight loss and weight loss maintenance: "Medical events are often reported as triggers for weight loss … Medical triggers may produce a teachable moment for weight control, resulting in better initial weight loss and long-term maintenance."

Weight maintenance gets easier

Studies show that weight loss maintenance gets easier the longer it is maintained. A 1998 study (Klem et al, Psychological symptoms in individuals successful at long-term maintenance of weight loss) found that there "was no evidence that long-term suppression of body weight is associated with psychological distress."

A 2000 study (Klem et al, Does weight loss maintenance become easier over time?) found: "Subjects who had maintained weight losses longer used fewer weight maintenance strategies and reported that less effort was required to diet and maintain weight and that less attention was required to maintain weight. … As duration increases, a shift in the balance between the effort and pleasure of weight maintenance may occur. This shift may increase the likelihood of continued maintenance."

A 2001 study (Wing et al, Successful weight loss maintenance) reported: "We found that in the National Weight Control Registry, successful long-term weight loss maintainers (average weight loss of 30 kg for an average of 5.5 years) share common behavioral strategies, including eating a diet low in fat, frequent self-monitoring of body weight and food intake, and high levels of regular physical activity. Weight loss maintenance may get easier over time. Once these successful maintainers have maintained a weight loss for 2-5 years, the chances of longer-term success greatly increase."

Joel Fuhrman MD

Born in New York, New York in 1953, Joel Fuhrman became a competitive figure skater, placing second in the U.S. National Pairs Championship in 1973. In 1973 he suffered a heel injury which disabled him for almost a year. He was advised to have surgery but instead consulted Herbert Shelton, a San Antonio naturopath who put him on a 46-day, water-only fast.

Recovering his health, Fuhrman decided to become a doctor specializing in nutrition medicine. Dr. Fuhrman assigned an ANDI (aggregate nutrient density index) score to common foods based on the micronutrients in the food (vitamins, minerals, antioxidants, phytochemicals) relative to the calories in the food (carbs, fat and protein). He created the formula H=N/C meaning your health equals the nutrient density of the foods you eat relative to the calories in the food.

Dr. Fuhrman recommends a nutrient-dense, plant-rich, "nutritarian" diet of primarily vegetables, fruit, beans, nuts and seeds with only limited amounts of animal foods. He uses the acronym G-BOMBS (greens, beans, onions, mushrooms, berries, seeds) for foods he recommends should be eaten daily.

Amazon provides the following recommendation for Dr. Fuhrman's bestseller, *Eat to Live: The Amazing Nutrient-Rich Program for Fast and Sustained Weight Loss*: "The Eat To Live 2011 revised edition includes updated scientific research supporting Dr. Fuhrman's revolutionary six-week plan… This is a book that will let you live longer, reduce your need for medications, and improve your health dramatically. It is a book that will change the way you want to eat.

Most importantly, if you follow the Eat To Live™ diet, you will lose weight faster than you ever thought possible."

Dr. Fuhrman's 2016 book, *The End of Heart Disease: The Eat to Live Plan to Prevent and Reverse Heart Disease*, argues for a nutritional approach to preventing and treating heart disease: "One of our country's leading experts in both preventive medicine and the science of food, Dr. Fuhrman speaks directly to readers everywhere who want to take control of their health and avoid taking medication or undergoing complicated, expensive, unnecessary, and often ineffective procedures or surgery. He asserts that the public is rarely informed by their doctors of the most effective options for treating high blood pressure, high cholesterol, and heart disease."

In addition to the books, audiobooks and videos in the list below, Dr. Fuhrman sponsors drfuhrman.com and can be seen in online videos by searching for "Joel Fuhrman".

Audiobooks by Joel Fuhrman

Eat For Health: Lose Weight, Keep It Off, Look Younger, Live Longer (2008)

Eat To Live: The Revolutionary Formula for Fast and Sustained Weight Loss (2012)

The End of Diabetes: The Eat To Live Plan to Prevent and Reverse Diabetes (2014)

The End of Dieting: How to Live For Life (2014)

The End of Heart Disease: The Eat To Live Plan to Prevent and Reverse Heart Disease (2016)

Books by Joel Fuhrman

Fasting and Eating For Health: A Medical Doctor's Program for Conquering Disease (1995)

Eat To Live: The Revolutionary Formula for Fast and Sustained Weight Loss (2003)

Disease-Proof Your Child: Feeding Kids Right (2005)

Eat For Health: Lose Weight, Keep It Off, Look Younger, Live Longer / 1- The Mind Makeover (2008)

Eat For Health: Lose Weight, Keep It Off, Look Younger, Live Longer / 2- The Body Makeover (2008)

Eat To Live: The Amazing Nutrient-Rich Program for Fast and Sustained Weight Loss (2009)
Super Immunity: The Essential Nutrition Guide for Boosting Our Body's Defenses ... (2011)
Eat For Health: Lose Weight, Keep It Off, Look Younger, Live Longer (2012)
Eat To Live: The Amazing Nutrient-Rich Program for Fast and Sustained Weight Loss (2012)
Nutritarian Handbook and ANDI Food Scoring Guide (2012)
Eat To Live Cookbook: 200 Delicious Nutrient-Rich Recipes for Fast and Sustained Weight Loss ... (2013)
The End of Diabetes: The Eat To Live Plan to Prevent And Reverse Diabetes (2013)
The End of Dieting: How to Live For Life (2014)
The End of Heart Disease: The Eat To Live Plan to Prevent and Reverse Heart Disease (2016)

DVDs with Joel Fuhrman

Get Healthy Now! [2005] by VegSource Interactive
Get Healthy Now! [2006] by VegSource Interactive
Get Healthy Now! [2007] by VegSource Interactive
Secrets to Healthy Cooking (2007)
Get Healthy Now! [2009] by VegSource.com
Get Healthy Now! [2010] by VegSource.com
Get Healthy Now! [2011] by VegSource.com

Michael Greger MD

Born in 1972 Michael Greger graduated from Cornell University School of Agriculture and Tufts University School of Medicine. Greger is a founder of the American College of Lifestyle Medicine. Dr. Greger, a vegan, is Director of Public Health and Animal Agriculture at The Humane Society of the United States. Greger started NutritionFacts.org, a non-profit website that has videos on hundreds of nutrition topics that are free to the public.

In 2015 Greger published *How Not to Die: Discover the Foods Scientifically Proven to Prevent and Reverse Disease*, a 576-page book that is also available as an audiobook. According to Amazon's review,

"From the physician behind the wildly popular website NutritionFacts.org, *How Not to Die* reveals the groundbreaking scientific evidence behind the only diet that can prevent and reverse many of the causes of disease-related death. The vast majority of premature deaths can be prevented through simple changes in diet and lifestyle. In *How Not to Die*, Dr. Michael Greger, the internationally-renowned nutrition expert, physician, and founder of NutritionFacts.org, examines the fifteen top causes of premature death in America…"

Reviews of *How Not to Die* are positive, including:

- "Michael Greger, M.D. scours the world's scholarly literature on nutrition for the most interesting, groundbreaking and practical new research. His work at NutritionFacts.org and in *How Not to Die* features the latest science on nutrition and health to show how to treat and prevent disease."--Joel Fuhrman MD, author of "Eat to Live"

- "The primary determinant of our health and well-being is what we eat and how we live. In this extraordinary and empowering book, Dr. Michael Greger explains why. Highly recommended."--Dean Ornish MD, author of "The Spectrum" and "Dr. Dean Ornish's Program for Reversing Heart Disease"

- "An absolute rhapsody of informational wisdom on how to achieve a life of health and longevity without disease."--Caldwell B. Esselstyn, Jr. MD, author of "Prevent and Reverse Heart Disease"

Audiobooks by Michael Greger

How Not To Die: Discover the Foods Scientifically Proven to Prevent and Reverse Disease (2015)
How Not to Diet: The Groundbreaking Science of Healthy Permanent Weight Loss (2019)

Books by Michael Greger

Carbophobia: The Scary Truth About America's Low-Carb Craze (2005)
Bird Flu: A Virus of Our Own Hatching (2006)

How Not To Die: Discover the Foods Scientifically Proven to Prevent and Reverse Disease (2015)
How Not to Diet: The Groundbreaking Science of Healthy Permanent Weight Loss (2019)

DVDs with Michael Greger

A River Of Waste: The Hazardous Truth About Factory Farms (2009)
PlantPure Nation: The Truth Is A Stubborn Thing. It Doesn't Go Away (2015)

Dean Ornish MD

Dean Ornish was born in 1953 in Dallas. He graduated first in his class from the University of Texas in Austin and obtained a medical degree from Baylor College of Medicine in Houston. He assisted with bypass surgeries as an intern at Massachusetts General Hospital but saw patients return to their old eating patterns and suffer further heart problems.

Dr. Ornish founded the Preventive Medicine Research Institute in Sausalito, California where he has conducted groundbreaking research on the use of diet, exercise, meditation and social support to treat coronary artery disease and prostate cancer and to lengthen telomeres. He convinced Medicare to pay for the cost of his heart disease treatment program for eligible Medicare patients.

Ornish recommends a diet high in vegetables, fruit and beans and low in refined grains, sugar and dairy. In an article in Scientific American he writes that "there is actually an emerging consensus among scientists and physicians who do research in nutrition about what constitutes an optimal way of eating. Although we always need more research, there is enough science now to guide us."

Audiobooks by Dean Ornish

The Spectrum: A Scientifically Proven Program to Feel Better, Live Longer, Lose Weight ... (2007)

Books by Dean Ornish

Stress, Diet, and Your Heart (1983)
Dr. Dean Ornish's Program for Reversing Heart Disease: The Only System Scientifically Proven ... (1990)
Eat More, Weigh Less: Dr. Dean Ornish's Life Choice Program for Losing Weight Safely ... (1993)
Everyday Cooking With Dr. Dean Ornish: 150 Easy, Low-Fat, High-Flavor Recipes (1996)
Love & Survival: The Scientific Basis for the Healing Power of Intimacy (1998)
Eat More, Weigh Less: Dr. Dean Ornish's Advantage Ten Program for Losing Weight Safely ... (2001)
The Spectrum: A Scientifically Proven Program to Feel Better, Live Longer, Lose Weight ... (2007)

DVDs with Dean Ornish

Love & Survival: Simple Choices, Powerful Changes (1998)
Breast Cancer: The Path of Wellness & Healing (2012)
The Connection (2014)

Caldwell Esselstyn MD

Caldwell Esselstyn Jr. was born in 1933 in New York City. He won a gold medal for rowing at the 1956 Olympics and graduated from Yale University and Western Reserve School of Medicine. Dr. Esselstyn was trained as a surgeon at the Cleveland Clinic, served as an army surgeon, was awarded the Bronze Star in Vietnam and has served on the Board of Governors of the Cleveland Clinic.

Esselstyn's book, *Prevent and Reverse Heart Disease*, documents his success at reversing coronary artery disease in his patients who followed a strict, low-fat, whole-food, plant-based diet. His diet allows vegetables, legumes, fruit and whole grains and prohibits animal and dairy foods, refined grains and all oils. Esselstyn works to bring cholesterol below 150 mg/dL and LDL cholesterol below 80 mg/dL.

President Bill Clinton had a quadruple heart bypass in 2004 and two angioplasty stents in 2010. In an interview, Clinton cited the work of Esselstyn, Ornish, T. Colin Campbell and Campbell's son for convincing him to adopt a plant-based diet which resulted in his loss of 24 pounds and plans to remain on the diet permanently.

Books by Caldwell Esselstyn

Prevent and Reverse Heart Disease: The Revolutionary, Scientifically Proven, Nutrition-Based Cure (2007)
Forks Over Knives: The Plant-Based Way to Health (2011)
Prevent and Reverse Heart Disease (2014)

DVDs with Caldwell Esselstyn

Get Healthy Now! [2005] by VegSource Interactive
Get Healthy Now! [2006] by VegSource Interactive
Get Healthy Now! [2007] by VegSource Interactive
Get Healthy Now! [2010] by VegSource Interactive
Forks Over Knives (2011)
Planeat (2011)
Prevent and Reverse Heart Disease: The DVD (2011)
Forks Over Knives: The Extended Interviews (2012)
Prevent and Reverse Heart Disease: Cooking Video (2015)

Chapter Three

Easy Meals

A Convenient Diet

This chapter describes the diet that I have usually followed when eating at home for almost 10 years now (since 2010). There have been some changes and a wide variety of other foods eaten at times.

Since I don't know your medical condition or history, I don't necessarily recommend this diet. I offer it only as a possible whole-food diet for your consideration. I've found the diet easy to shop for, relatively inexpensive, quick and easy to prepare and quick and easy to clean up after.

Many diets fail because they are not as quick and convenient as alternatives. Grocery store convenience foods and restaurants have made eating a diet of animal and processed foods very convenient.

Grocery store convenience foods became popular following World War II. Candy, soft drinks and juices, frozen pizza and potato products, breakfast cereals, sliced bread, lunch meats and cheeses, canned soups, corn and potato chips, cookies, crackers, and ice cream are typical convenience foods. These foods are often high in calories and low in nutrition and often contain added fats, oils, refined flour, sugar and salt.

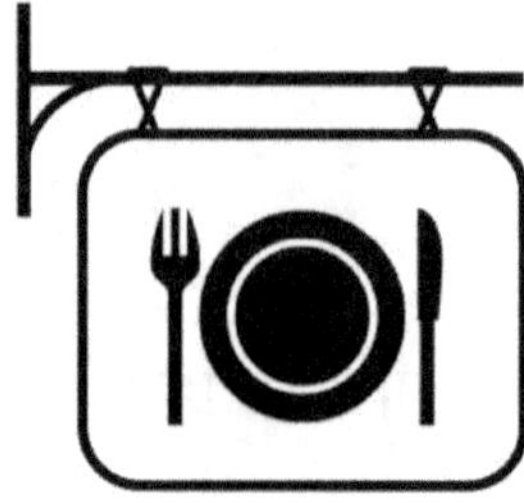

Along with the growth of convenient processed foods, restaurant eating has become much more popular. A report by the USDA Economic Research Service found that food-away-from-home (restaurants, take-out and home delivery) increased from 26% of food spending in 1970 to 43% in 2012. Pizza from a pizza delivery company, fast food meals from a drive-through and restaurant meals are all very convenient.

While food-away-from-home is convenient, it's often unhealthy. The USDA reports that food-away-from-home is lower in dietary fiber and higher in saturated fat and sodium contributing to "obesity, heart disease, stroke, cancer, diabetes, osteoarthritis, and other health conditions".

Many people find that a healthy, whole-food diet requires spending a good deal of time shopping for produce that quickly spoils, keeping lots of fresh ingredients on hand, preparing complicated recipes, and time-consuming kitchen clean-up.

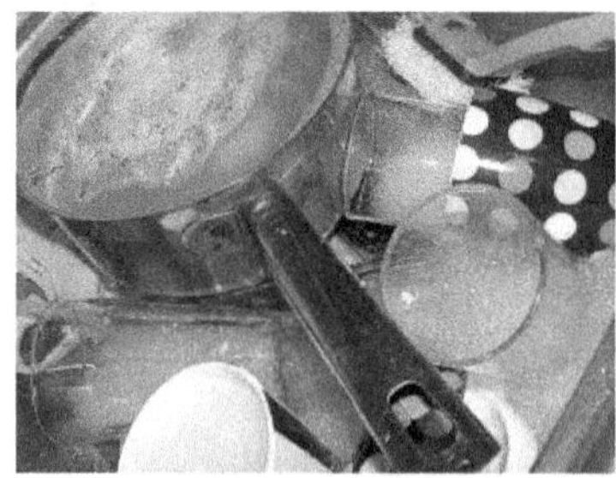

For people who don't want to spend a lot of time in the kitchen, the modern diet of convenience foods and restaurant fare seems like the only practical alternative. When time is short and easier alternatives exist, it can be hard to stick with a healthy diet. People sometimes feel that they have no choice but to eat the way they do.

However healthy meals can be fast and easy - easy to shop for, easy to prepare and easy to clean up.

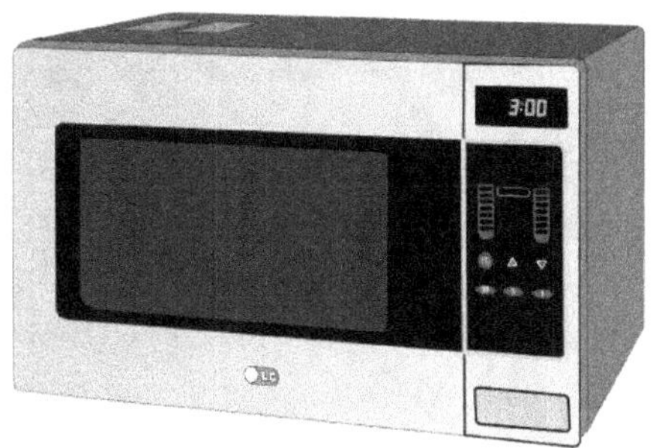

Two modern inventions make eating healthy meals practical and convenient: Frozen vegetables and microwave ovens.

Frozen vegetables and fruit are great for convenience since they come washed and cut, last a long time without spoiling, have little waste, are usually flash frozen within hours of being picked, and are often more nutritious than fresh which may be eaten many days after being picked.

A single bowl and spoon are all the tableware needed for many meals. Fresh and frozen foods are quickly combined and microwaved, making preparation and clean-up fast and easy.

An Unvarying Diet

The National Weight Control Registry (NWCR), the study of strategies used by members who have lost significant weight and kept it off long-term, has found that adopting a meal plan that stays the same day after day makes it easier to eat a healthy diet until it becomes automatic and habitual.

An article in **Today's Dietitian** "The Seven Secrets of Successful Weight Loss" says the NWCR strategy of eating the same thing every day works because food decisions become routine, food temptations are minimized, self-control and self-discipline are encouraged, and the ability to persevere with the diet is increased.

The article goes on to say that those who follow a consistent meal pattern tend to weigh less than those who follow "an inconsistent, random, or chaotic meal pattern."

Dr. Michael Roisin in his DVD *You on a Diet* (2006, 100 minutes) distills essential action steps for successful weight loss:

- Walk 30 minutes a day,
- Restock your kitchen (discard simple sugars, refined flour, saturated and trans fats); and,
- Automate (make it easy on yourself by avoiding too many choices and eating roughly the same thing each day).

By simplifying your daily meal plan, food decisions become automatic and effortless. Rearrange your kitchen and food supply so that eating the same healthy foods every day is simple, quick and convenient and in time automatic, routine and habitual. When you get up in the morning, you don't agonize over what to eat for breakfast. Everything is on hand and convenient.

Find a daily meal plan that suits you and that you can follow until it becomes your normal way of eating. Focus on healthy, high-fiber foods:

- Fruit
- Vegetables
- Beans and lentils
- Nuts and seeds
- Oatmeal and other whole grains
- Vinegar and spices
- Water, coffee and tea.

Avoid processed foods (i.e., foods with added fats, added oils, added sugars, refined grains, and processed meats). Limit animal foods (e.g., meat, eggs, cheese and milk).

Keep your meal plan simple and consistent from day to day until it becomes your normal way of eating. After a healthy diet becomes routine, add variety to your diet by adding and substituting different fruit, vegetables, beans, nuts, seeds, grains and spices.

As new information becomes available about the nutritional content of foods, changes will be warranted. See for example a video by Dr. Michael Greger about the cancer fighting power of various vegetables. Search online for "greger #1 anticancer vegetable".

Kitchen Equipment

Below are some items that I've found helpful for preparing food.

Microwave oven Other heating methods are possible but none is as quick and convenient as a microwave oven. A 2009 study in the Journal of Food Science titled "Influence of cooking methods on antioxidant activity of vegetables" found boiling among the worst methods for nutrient loss and microwaving among the best. Search online for "greger best cooking method" for a short video on cooking methods.

Be careful setting cooking time on a microwave. Setting the time at 30 minutes intending 3 minutes can result in a fire in the microwave.

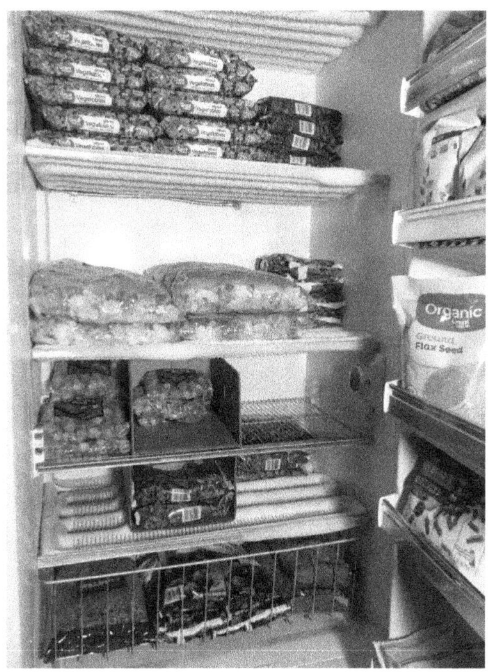

Separate freezer A stand-alone freezer for vegetables, blueberries, walnuts, almonds, flaxseed, chia seeds and other items is not essential but makes food storage easier.

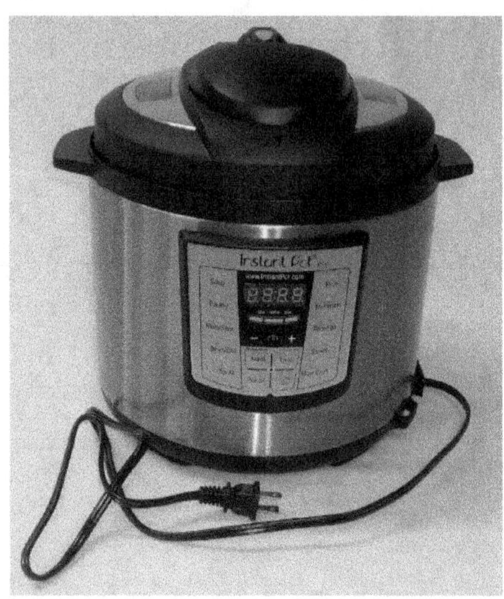

Pressure cooker The 6-quart Instant Pot shown is useful for cooking many foods. I use it mostly for beans and lentils. Unlike conventional pressure cookers the heat turns off automatically at the set time. A pressure cooker is optional. Canned beans and lentils are another option.

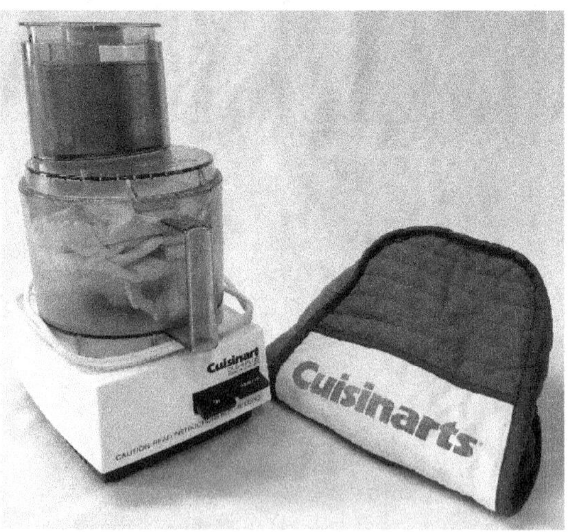

Food processor A food processor is optional but useful for slicing red cabbage.

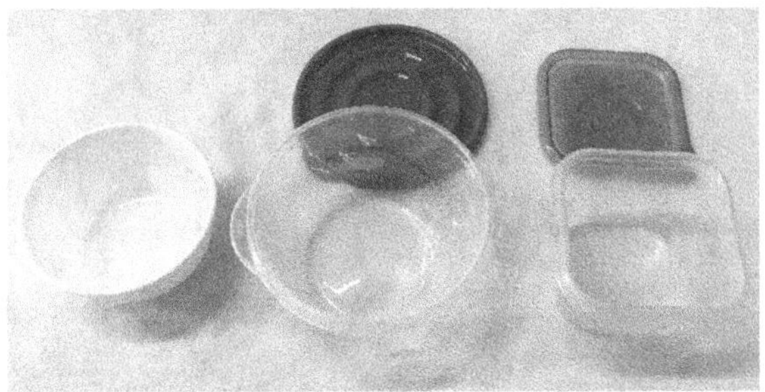

Microwave-safe bowls Corelle Livingware glass 28 oz. (3.5 cup) soup bowls, thin, light, microwave-safe bowls, don't get excessively hot in the microwave. About $5.00 at Walmart. A single bowl and spoon suffices for most meals, making clean up quick and easy without needing to run a dishwasher.

Plastic containers Rubbermaid 6.2-cup bowl used for sliced red cabbage. Ziploc's 4-cup square storage containers used for freezing beans and lentils prepared in a pressure cooker. Also used for frozen blueberries and chopped red onions.

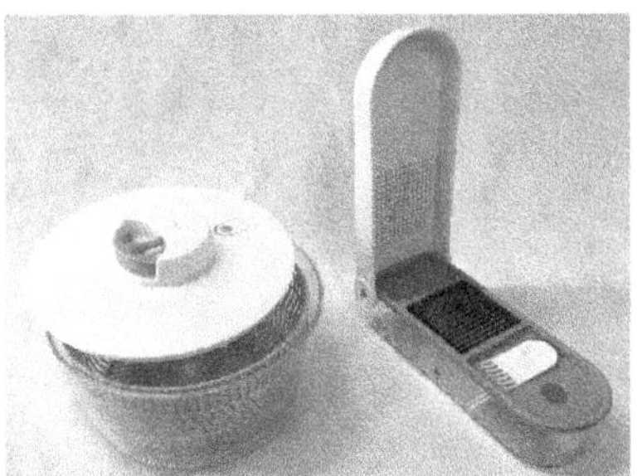

Salad spinner For rinsing, drying and storing leafy greens in your refrigerator.

Onion chopper Useful for chopping red onions. Search online for "greger carrots vs baby carrots" for a comparison of red, yellow and white onions.

The food chopper shown (about $17 at Walmart) makes chopping onions easier. Cut the top and bottom off of the onion. Cut the onion into 4 parts (perpendicular to the top and bottom cuts). Remove the paper-like layer of the onion. Cut each fourth in half. Place a section on the grate and slam the lid very hard.

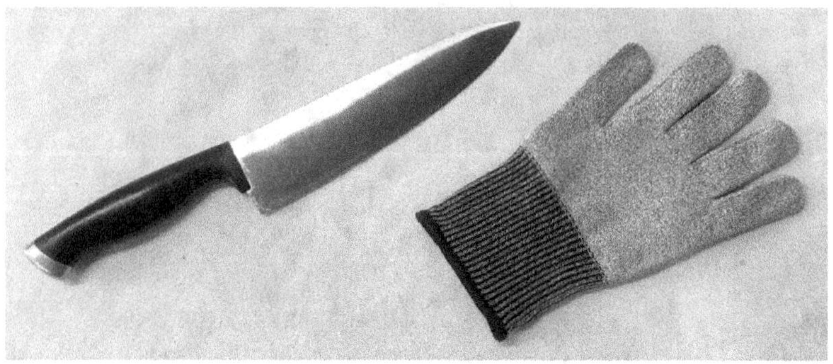

Chef's knife For cutting red cabbage and red onions.
Cut resistant glove For holding onions, cabbage and other vegetables when cutting with a chef's knife.

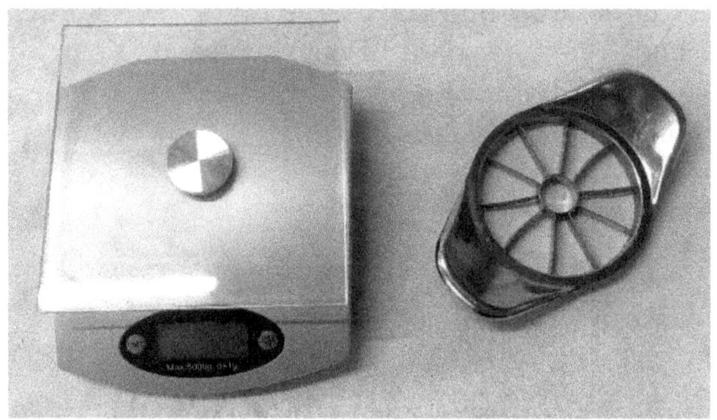

Scale For measuring food and keeping a food journal.
Apple slicer

The following sections provide examples of foods to have on hand.

Frozen Food

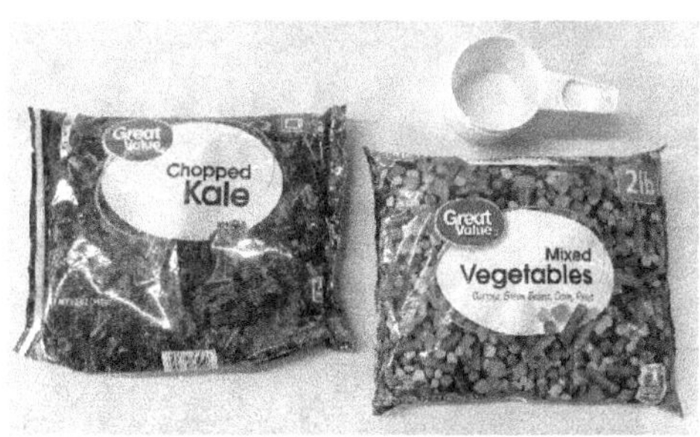

Chopped kale Walmart, 12 oz.
Mixed vegetables Walmart, 2 lb., 3/4 cup scoop kept in the bag.

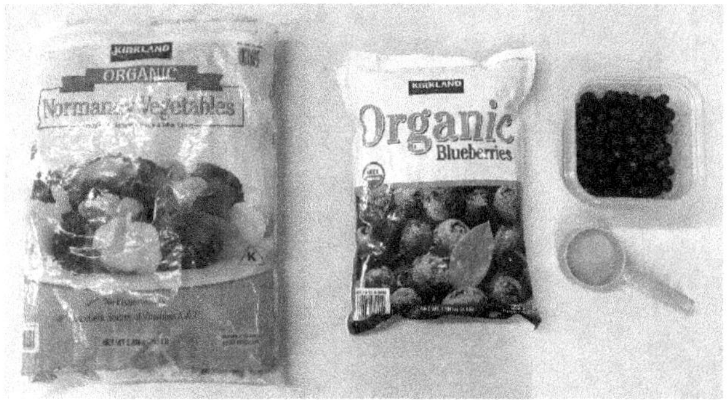

Normandy vegetables (broccoli, cauliflower and carrots) Costco, 5.5 lb. Normandy vegetables also available at Walmart.

Blueberries Costco, 3 lb., 1/3 cup scoop kept in the plastic container.

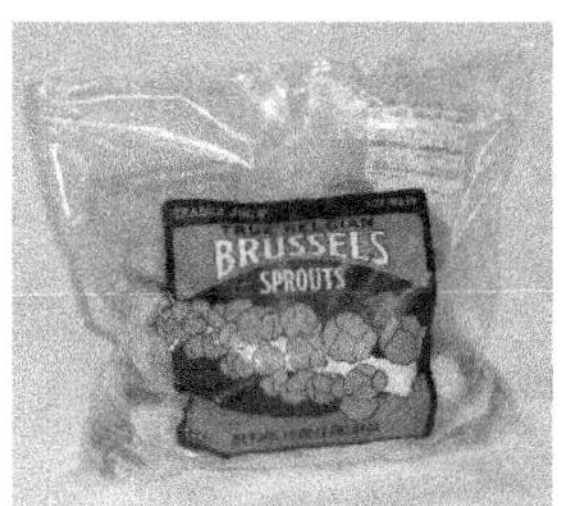

Brussels sprouts Trader Joe's, 1 lb.

Produce

Apples Search online for "greger antioxidant content of 300 foods" for a video on the top antioxidant foods.
Bananas
Oranges
Red onions
Red cabbage

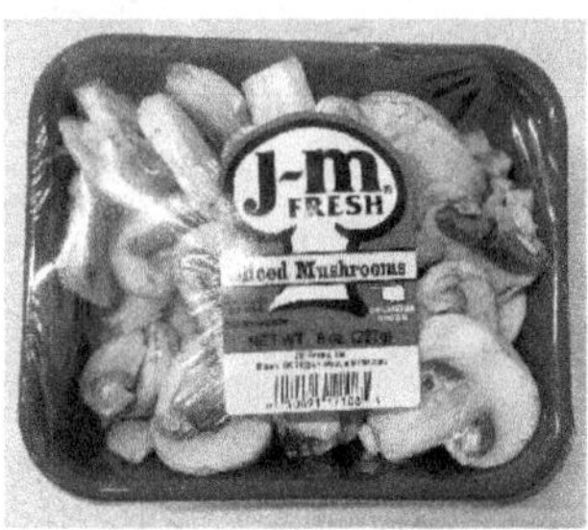

Mushrooms Until recently mushrooms were available as a frozen food at Walmart. Fresh is a slightly more expensive and less convenient alternative. Eat mushrooms cooked, not raw. Avoid canned mushrooms that are high in salt.

Nuts and Seeds

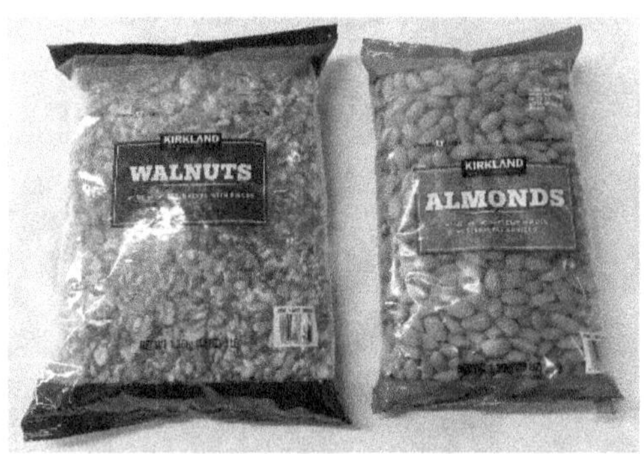

Walnuts Costco, 3 lb. Search online for "greger which nut fights cancer better?" for a video.
Almonds Costco, 3 lb.

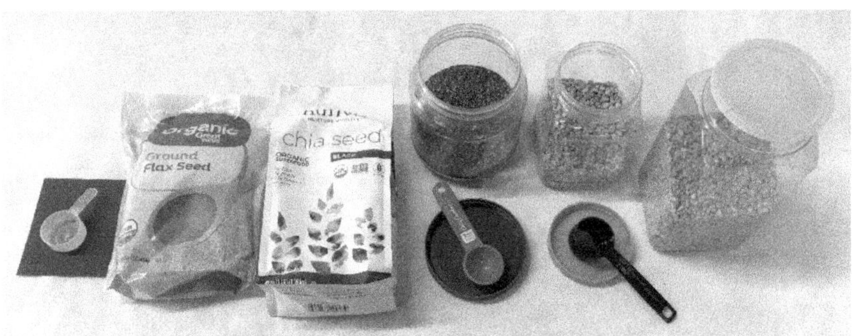

Ground flaxseed Walmart, 1 lb. Store flaxseed in freezer to preserve freshness. 25 cc (1.67 oz. tablespoon) scoop kept in the bag.

Chia seeds Costco, 2 lb. Search online for "greger flax seeds vs. chia seeds" for a short video. 1 tablespoon scoop kept in the container.

Sunflower seeds Sprouts Farmers Market, bulk sales. Two tablespoon scoop kept in the smaller container.

Beverages

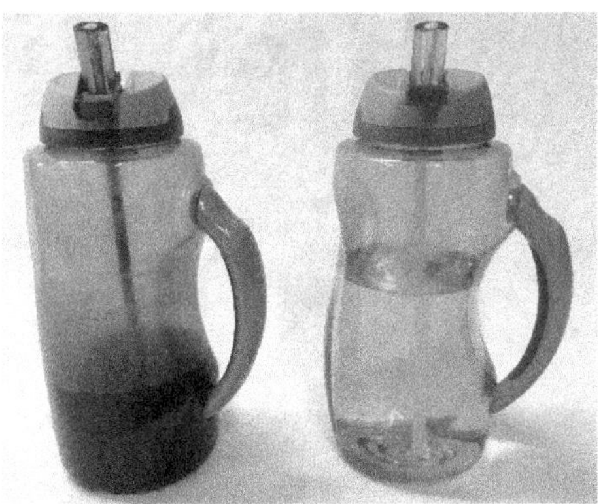

Coffee and water Instant coffee consumed cold. 63 oz, mugs available at Walmart. See Wikipedia coffee article for studies of the benefits and risks of coffee.

Tea Often green tea, but search online for "greger better than green tea" for a short video on the antioxidant power of hibiscus tea.

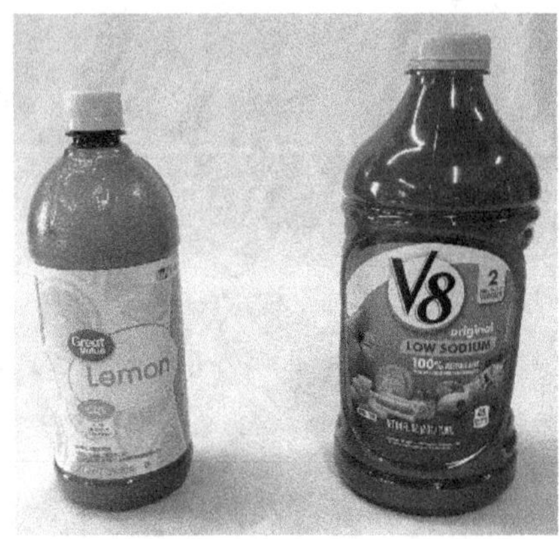

Lemon juice Walmart, 32 oz. For a short video on lemons and cancer, search online for "greger which fruit fights cancer better".
Vegetable juice Walmart, 64 oz. Low sodium.

Other Food

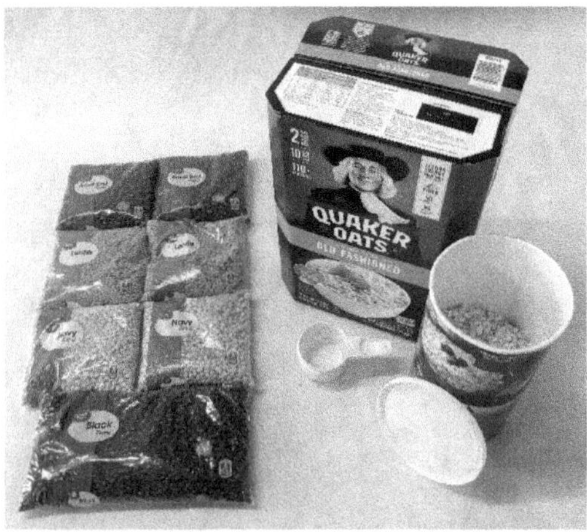

Beans and lentils Walmart, 1 and 2 lb. bags. Search online for "greger increased lifespan from beans" for a video.
Oatmeal Costco, 10 lb. Ten-pound box contains 2 five-pound bags. Two cylindrical containers hold the contents of a five-pound bag. Half-cup scoop kept in the container.

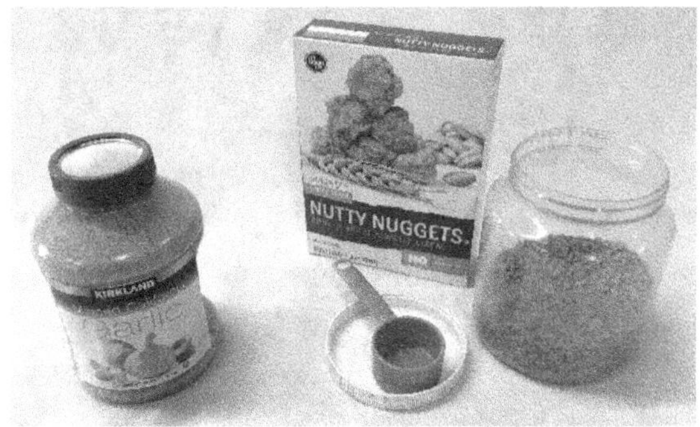

Minced garlic Costco, 3 lb.

Nutty Nuggets cereal Kroger, 20.5 oz., 1/4 cup scoop kept in the container.

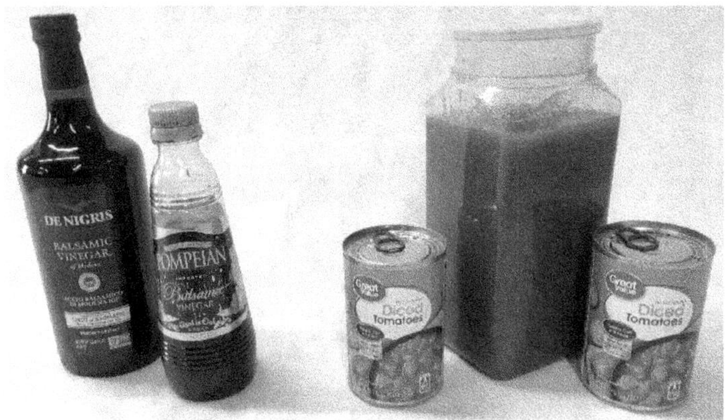

Balsamic vinegar Walmart, 33.8 oz. and 16 oz. Vinegars are a way to flavor food without the oil, sugar and salt of many salad dressings. Search online for "greger vinegar" for several short videos.

Diced tomatoes Walmart, 14.5 oz. No salt added. Five cans of tomatoes are poured into the larger container for easier handling. Clean container when empty to avoid spoilage.

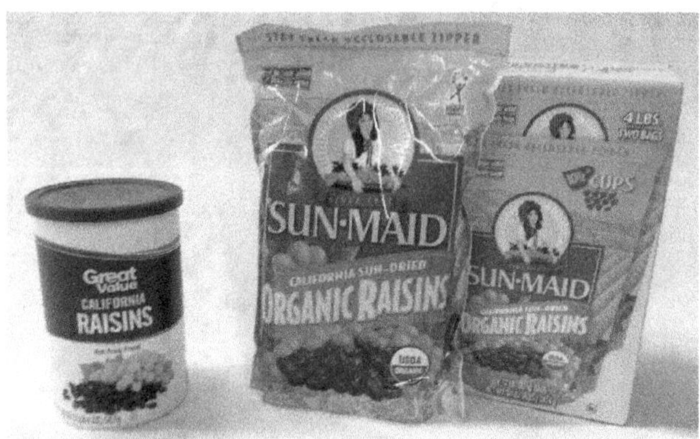

Raisins Costco, 2 lb. bags.

Spices

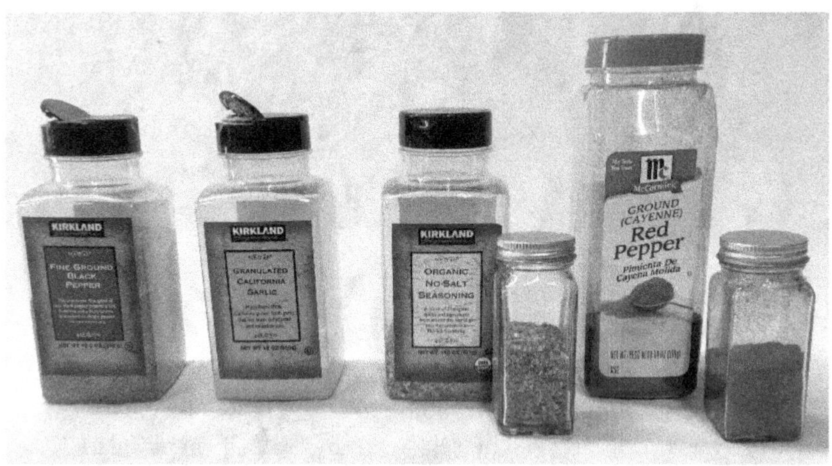

Black pepper Costco, 12.3 oz. Fine or course ground.

Granulated garlic Costco, 18 oz. Search online for "greger #1 anticancer vegetable".

No-salt seasonings Costco, 14.5 oz. Smaller container for easier handling.

Cayenne pepper Costco, 14 oz. If you like spicy food. Smaller container for easier handling.

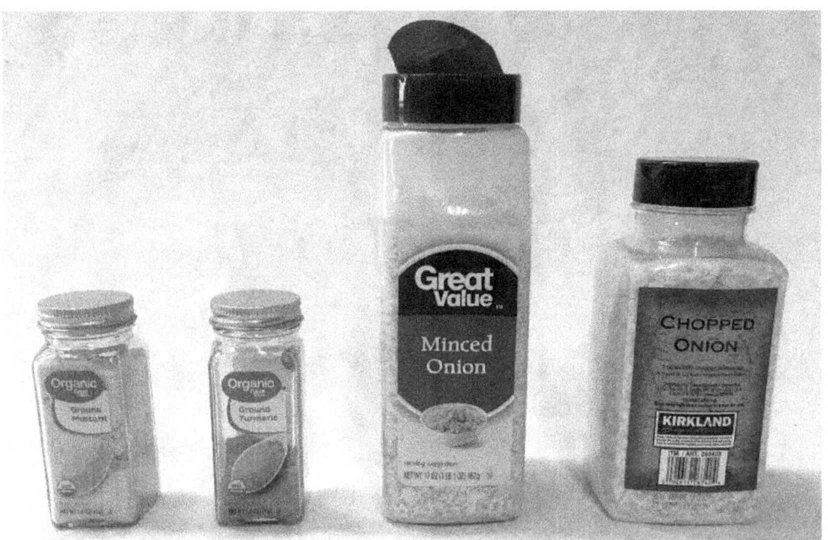

Ground mustard Walmart, 1.6 oz. Search online for "greger mustard" for Second Strategy to Cooking Broccoli.

Turmeric Walmart, 1.8 oz. Search online for "greger turmeric" for videos including benefits and risks.

Dried onions Walmart (Minced Onion) 17 oz. or Costco (Chopped Onion) 11.7 oz.

Oatmeal Bowl

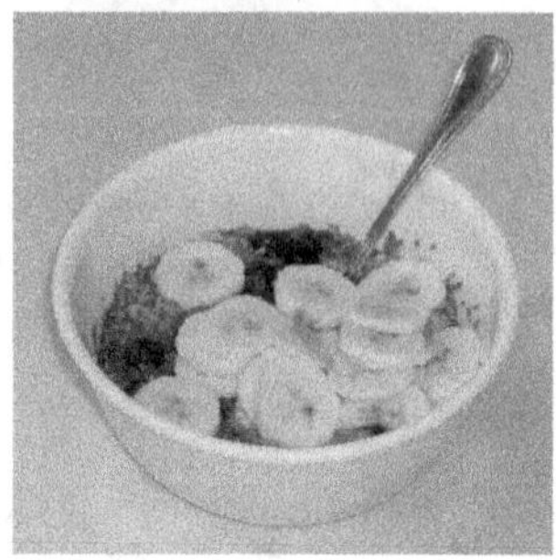

Add:

- One-half cup of old-fashioned rolled oats
- One-half cup of frozen blueberries
- One tablespoon of ground flaxseed
- One tablespoon of chia seeds
- About a cup of water

Heat in your microwave (about 3 minutes for 2 bowls). While the oatmeal is cooking, peel a banana to be sliced and added to the cooked oatmeal.

The chia seeds add additional fiber and can absorb over ten times their weight in water for additional bulk and satiety. Fiber, carbs, fat and protein in the table below are in grams (1/28 ounce). Sodium is in micrograms (1/1000 gram).

Oatmeal bowl	amt	cals	fibr	carb	fat	protn	sodm
oatmeal	½ cup dry	154	4	27	3	5	2
blueberries	½ cup frozen	59	3	14	1	0	1
flaxseed	1 tablespoon	38	2	2	3	1	2
chia seeds	1 tablespoon	49	3	4	3	2	2
banana	½ medium	52	2	14	0	1	1
		352	14	61	10	9	8

Cabbage Bowl

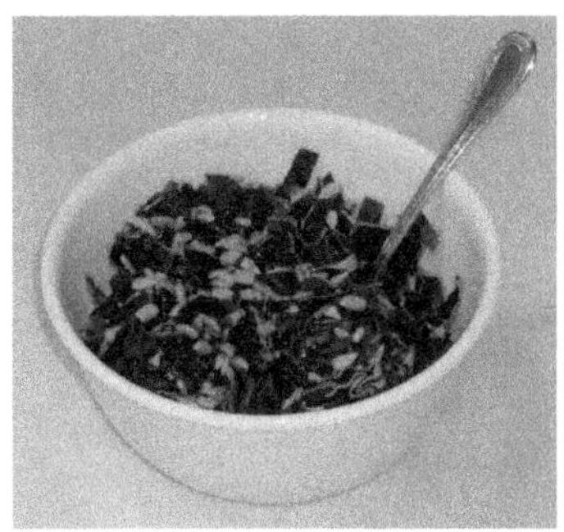

Add:

- 6 oz. (1.5 cups) of frozen mixed vegetables
- A small amount (1 oz.) of frozen sliced mushrooms
- 3 oz. (1.5 cups) of frozen chopped kale
- 1 oz. (1/4 cup) of Grape Nuts or similar grain cereal
- 3 oz. (1/2 cup) of beans or lentils

Heat in your microwave (about 4 minutes for one bowl). While the bowl is cooking, set out sliced cabbage, sunflower seeds and balsamic vinegar.

Add a large handful of sliced red cabbage (3 oz.). Top with a tablespoon of sunflower seeds and about 2 tablespoons of balsamic vinegar.

Search online for "greger superfood bargains" for the antioxidant power of red (aka purple) cabbage, and "greger vinegar" for several vinegar videos.

Cabbage bowl	amt	cals	fibr	carb	fat	protn	sodm
mixed vegetables	6 ounces	142	5	27	1	5	48
mushrooms	1 ounce	8	1	2	0	1	1
kale	3 ounces	26	2	4	0	2	13
grape nuts	1 ounce	98	3	24	1	3	144
black beans	3 ounces	112	7	20	1	8	1
red cabbage	3 ounces	26	2	6	0	1	23
sunflower seeds	1 tablespoon	51	1	2	4	2	1
balsamic vinegar	2 tablespoons	28	0	5	0	0	7
		491	21	90	7	22	238

Broccoli Bowl

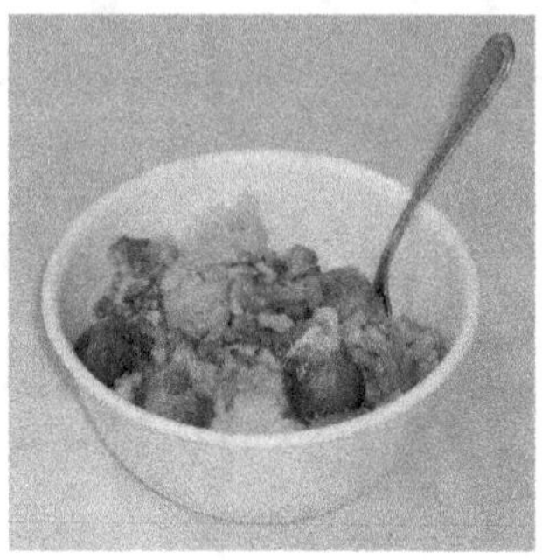

Add:

- A 10-ounce mix of frozen broccoli florets, cauliflower and carrots.
- 3 oz. of frozen Brussels sprouts (about 5 to 9 depending on their size)

Heat in your microwave (about 6 minutes for one bowl). While the bowl is cooking, set out walnuts and ground mustard seed.

Top the heated bowl with a half-ounce of walnuts (seven walnut halves) and a sprinkling (about one-quarter teaspoon) of ground mustard seeds to activate the cancer-fighting sulforaphane in the broccoli, cauliflower and Brussels sprouts.

Nuts or seeds are eaten with each of the bowls to improve absorption of vegetable nutrients.

Search online for "greger mustard" for his Second Strategy to Cooking Broccoli video for the reason to use ground mustard seeds.

Drink a cup of vegetable juice with about an ounce of lemon juice added. There is evidence that broccoli and tomatoes interact favorably.

Broccoli bowl	amt	cals	fibr	carb	fat	protn	sodm
broccoli	4 ounces	32	3	6	0	4	12
cauliflower	3 ounces	16	2	3	0	1	15
carrots	3 ounces	32	3	7	1	0	50
brussels sprouts	3 ounces	36	4	7	0	3	13
walnuts	½ ounce	93	1	2	9	2	0
		209	13	25	10	10	90

Dinner Bowl

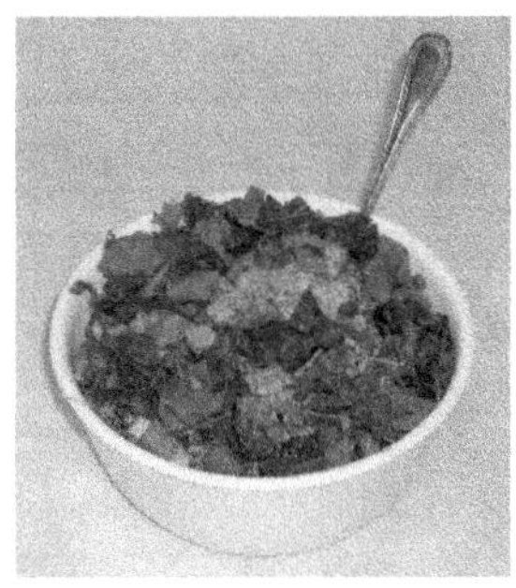

Add:
- 6 oz. (1.5 cups) of frozen mixed vegetables
- 3 oz. (1.5 cups) of frozen chopped kale
- 1 oz. (1/4 cup) of Grape Nuts or similar grain cereal
- 3 oz. (1/2 cup) of beans or lentils
- 2 tablespoons of dried onions
- One cup of diced tomatoes

Heat in your microwave (about 7 minutes for 2 bowls).

While the bowls are cooking, set out:
- Chopped red onions
- Minced garlic
- Almonds
- Turmeric
- Black pepper
- No-salt seasoning mix
- Granulated garlic

To each heated bowl add 2 oz. of chopped red onions, an ounce of minced garlic, 11 almonds (1/2 oz.), and a sprinkling of turmeric, black pepper, no-salt seasoning mix and granulated garlic. Add cayenne pepper if desired.

Dinner bowl	amt	cals	fibr	carb	fat	protn	sodm
mixed vegetables	6 ounces	142	5	27	1	5	48
kale	3 ounces	26	2	4	0	2	13
grape nuts	1 ounce	98	3	24	1	3	144
lentils	3 ounces	99	5	17	0	8	2
dried onions	2 tablespoons	60	3	14	0	2	12
tomatoes	1 cup diced	77	5	18	1	4	20
red onions	2 ounces	23	1	5	0	1	2
minced garlic	1 ounce	28	0	6	0	0	0
almonds	½ ounce (11)	82	2	3	7	3	0
		635	26	118	10	28	261

Other ingredients sometimes added to the bowls include:

- Fresh greens (e.g., kale, parsley, arugula, cilantro, etc. kept in the refrigerator in a salad spinner)
- Avocado
- Beets
- Sweet potatoes and yams
- Potatoes
- Apple cider vinegar
- Hot peppers
- Sweet peppers
- Hot and mild salsas
- Horseradish
- Cumin
- Brown rice
- Wild rice
- Quinoa
- Buckwheat
- Millet
- Couscous.

Other Quick Meals

The meals described above are quick and easy with only a bowl and spoon to clean. There are other ways to cook healthy food that are also quick and inexpensive. Jeff Novick, a dietician, chef and speaker has produced a series of DVDs on healthy, plant-based cooking entitled *Fast Food* that are available from Amazon, Vegsource.com and some libraries.

Volume 1 of *Fast Food* describes how to prepare Indian potato stew with curry, Mexican beans and rice, Italian pasta primavera, Longevity soup, and New Orleans jambalaya by varying 5 basic ingredients: canned tomatoes, canned beans, frozen vegetables, a starch (e.g., potato, corn, pasta, sweet potato, rice) and a store-bought spice mix. Daily per person meal cost is estimated at under $4.00. Jeff Novick's other videos on how to read nutrition labels, prepare vegan burgers and fries and understand the calorie density of foods are also recommended.

Chapter Four

Exercise

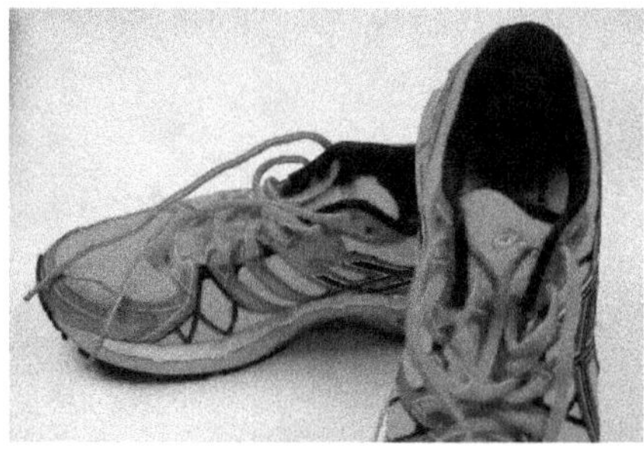

WHO and CDC Recommendations

The World Health Organization recommends for adults 18 to 64:
- 150 minutes per week of **moderate-intensity** aerobic exercise, **or**
- 75 minutes per week of **vigorous-intensity** aerobic exercise, **and**
- Muscle-strengthening exercises of major muscle groups 2 or more days a week.

The aerobic exercise should be "in bouts of at least 10 minutes duration".

According to the CDC, regular physical activity "can help:
- Control your weight
- Reduce your risk of cardiovascular disease
- Reduce your risk for type 2 diabetes and metabolic syndrome
- Reduce your risk of some cancers
- Strengthen your bones and muscles
- Improve your mental health and mood
- Improve your ability to do daily activities and prevent falls, if you're an older adult
- Increase your chances of living longer"

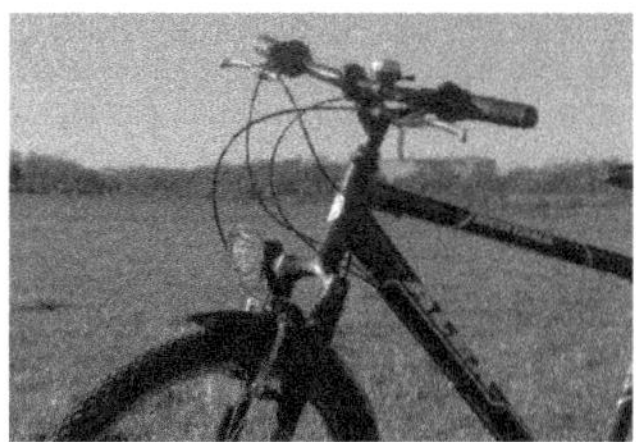

Examples of **moderate-intensity** aerobics: brisk walking (3 miles per hour), bicycling under 10 miles per hour, doubles tennis, ballroom dancing, and gardening.

Examples of **vigorous-intensity** aerobics: jogging, bicycling over 10 miles per hour, singles tennis, aerobics dancing, hiking uphill, and jumping rope.

Examples of muscle-strengthening exercises: lifting weights, push-ups, sit-ups, chin-ups.

For an isometric exercise that takes only 90 seconds, search online for "youtube 90 second isometric workout".

Exercise Mortality Studies

A 2011 meta-analysis analyzed 22 studies to determine the relationship between physical activity such as walking and all-cause mortality. The 22 studies included 977,925 men and women.

The study found that exercising 150 minutes a week (equivalent to 30 minutes/day, 5 days/week) was associated with a 19% reduction in mortality risk compared to non-exercisers. Increasing exercise to 7 hours/week was associated with a 24% reduction in mortality risk.

The study concluded that "Being physically active reduces the risk of all-cause mortality. The largest benefit was found from moving from no activity to low levels of activity, but even at high levels of activity benefits accrue from additional activity."

A 2015 meta-analysis analyzed 9 cohort studies with 122,417 men and women over the age of 60. The participants were divided into 4 groups: (1) Those who didn't exercise, (2) A low exercise group who exercised but failed to meet recommendations, (3) A group near the range of current recommendations, (4) A group who significantly exceeded current recommendations

Compared to those who didn't exercise, the low exercise group was associated with a 22% reduction in mortality risk, the middle exercise group with a 28% reduction in mortality risk and the high exercise group with a 35% reduction in mortality risk.

To your health. All the best.

© 2020 Revised: 1-26-2020